LOW CARB DIET FOOD LIST

The Complete Ingredient list and Food to Avoid for Low Carb Diet

Harley W. Norman

Table of Contents

Introduction to Low Carb Eating

In the bustling city of Everwell, where the pace of life never slows, Sarah found herself at a crossroads. Once an avid marathon runner, her life had taken a turn towards endless workdays and quick, unhealthy meals. The reflection in the mirror began to tell a story she hardly recognized, filled with fatigue and a health warning from her doctor. It was during one such evening, scrolling through her phone for a semblance of a solution, that she stumbled upon an ad for a book: "Low Carb Diet Food List"

The title resonated with her, a beacon of hope amidst her health concerns. The book promised not just a diet but a transformation towards a healthier, more vibrant life. Intrigued and slightly skeptical, Sarah decided to give it a chance, unaware of how much her life was about to change.

From the moment she turned the first page, "Low Carb Diet Food List" was unlike any other health book she had read. It wasn't just about cutting carbs or losing weight; it was a journey into understanding her body's needs and how food could be both nourishing and enjoyable. The introduction shared stories of individuals just like her, who had transformed their lives by making simple, sustainable changes to their diet.

As she delved into the chapters, Sarah discovered a comprehensive list of foods she could enjoy, from leafy greens and succulent berries to rich nuts and savory meats. The book demystified the low carb diet, explaining not only the 'what' but the 'why' behind each food choice. It was written with a warmth and wisdom that made Sarah feel supported and understood, not judged.

Meal planning became an adventure rather than a chore. Sarah experimented with recipes from the book, finding joy in cooking and satisfaction in the flavors. The Quick and Easy Low Carb Breakfast Ideas revolutionized her mornings, offering energy and no mid-morning crashes. Dinners were a time to savor the delicious Low Carb Dinners, which even her skeptical family enjoyed.

What truly set this book apart was its approach to challenges and setbacks. The chapters on Overcoming Challenges and Advanced Low Carb Strategies provided Sarah with tools to navigate cravings, social events, and the inevitable plateau. It wasn't just a diet; it was a lifestyle change that the book was guiding her through, step by patient step.

Three months into her journey, Sarah felt reborn. The weight loss was significant, yes, but what mattered more was the return of her energy, the clarity of her mind, and a newfound joy in movement.

She had rediscovered her love for running, not as a way to burn calories, but as a celebration of what her body could do.

Why should you buy "Low Carb Diet Food List"? Because it's not just a book; it's a companion on your journey to a healthier life. It understands the struggles, celebrates the victories, and guides you through every step with wisdom and compassion. For Sarah, it wasn't just about the low carb foods she learned to incorporate into her diet; it was about transforming her life in a way she never thought possible.

So, if you find yourself at a crossroads, looking for a path to better health and vitality, let "Low Carb Diet Food List" be your guide. It's more than a diet; it's a new beginning.

What is a Low Carb Diet?

A low carb diet focuses on minimizing the intake of carbohydrates, primarily found in sugary foods, pasta, and bread, to promote weight loss and improve overall health. By reducing carbs, the body is forced to use alternative fuel sources, namely fats, which leads to the production of ketones in the liver. These ketones serve as an efficient energy source for the body and brain, facilitating weight loss, reducing blood sugar and insulin levels, and providing a steady energy flow without the peaks and crashes associated with high carb meals.

This diet emphasizes the consumption of proteins, healthy fats, and vegetables, steering clear of processed foods and high-carb grains. Beginners are introduced to a food list that prioritizes leafy greens like spinach and kale, cruciferous vegetables such as broccoli and cauliflower, and low glycemic index fruits like berries. Proteins are sourced from lean meats, fish, eggs, and plant-based alternatives, ensuring muscle mass is maintained while fat stores are metabolized.

Healthy fats play a crucial role, derived from sources like avocados, nuts, seeds, and olive oil, supporting cell structure and hormone production without spiking blood sugar levels. This balanced approach to eating encourages a more mindful relationship with food, focusing on nutrient density and satiety rather than caloric content alone.

, navigating a low carb diet can initially seem daunting due to the widespread prevalence of carbs in the standard diet. However, the transition becomes more manageable with a comprehensive food list that outlines permissible foods, offering a variety of options to keep meals interesting and satisfying. This diet is not just about restriction but about discovering the vast array of foods that naturally support a low carb lifestyle.

By adhering to a low carb diet, individuals may experience significant health benefits, including improved cholesterol levels, reduced risk of heart disease, and better control over diabetes and insulin resistance. It also promotes mental clarity and energy levels, combating the sluggishness often associated with high carb diets.

Adopting a low carb diet doesn't necessitate a complete overhaul of eating habits overnight. Beginners are encouraged to start gradually, reducing carb intake while increasing their intake of vegetables, proteins, and fats to find a sustainable balance. This methodical approach helps to mitigate potential side effects like the keto flu, making the transition smoother.

In essence, a low carb diet offers a pathway to better health and well-being, focusing on whole, unprocessed foods. It's a lifestyle change that goes beyond mere weight loss, advocating for a holistic approach to nutrition that can be tailored to individual needs, preferences, and health goals. The Low Carb Diet Food List serves as a foundational guide, equipping newcomers with the knowledge to embark on this nutritional journey with confidence.

Benefits of Low Carb Eating

Low carb eating is a nutritional approach that has garnered significant attention for its potential to promote weight loss, enhance mental clarity, and improve overall health. By focusing on foods that are low in carbohydrates, individuals can shift their body's primary energy source from glucose to stored fats, a process known as ketosis. This metabolic state is associated with numerous health benefits, including a reduction in blood sugar and insulin levels, which can help manage and prevent diabetes. Carbohydrates, especially refined ones, tend to spike blood sugar levels, leading to increased insulin secretion. Over time, this can lead to insulin resistance, a precursor to type 2 diabetes. By reducing carbohydrate intake, low carb diets can mitigate these spikes, offering a preventive measure against the development of insulin resistance and diabetes.

Moreover, low carb eating emphasizes the consumption of nutrient-dense foods such as lean proteins, healthy fats, and fibrous vegetables, which can lead to improved satiety. This natural reduction in appetite can significantly decrease overall calorie intake, facilitating weight loss without the need for calorie counting or portion control. Many people find this aspect of low carb diets appealing, as it allows for a more intuitive approach to eating while still achieving weight loss goals.

Another notable benefit is the impact on cardiovascular health. By replacing dietary carbohydrates with healthy fats, individuals can see improvements in heart disease risk factors, including reductions in triglycerides, a type of fat found in the blood, and increases in high-density lipoprotein (HDL) cholesterol, often referred to as 'good' cholesterol. These changes can lead to a decreased risk of heart disease, particularly when the diet focuses on heart-healthy fats such as those from avocados, nuts, seeds, and olive oil.

Low carb eating can also have a positive effect on mental health and cognitive function. Fluctuations in blood sugar levels can affect brain function, leading to mood swings, fatigue, and difficulty concentrating. By stabilizing blood sugar through a low carb diet, individuals may experience improved focus, stable energy levels throughout the day, and enhanced mood stability. This aspect is particularly beneficial for individuals with demanding lifestyles or those prone to energy dips and mood fluctuations.

Additionally, for people suffering from specific health conditions such as polycystic ovary syndrome (PCOS), epilepsy, and metabolic syndrome, low carb diets have been shown to offer therapeutic benefits. For example, reducing carbohydrate intake can help manage PCOS symptoms by improving insulin sensitivity, while ketogenic diets, a strict form of low carb eating, have been used for decades to reduce epileptic seizures in individuals for whom medication is ineffective.

Incorporating a variety of low carb foods into one's diet can also lead to an increased intake of antioxidants and other nutrients found in vegetables and fruits permitted within these dietary guidelines. These nutrients play crucial roles in protecting the body against oxidative stress and inflammation, underlying factors in numerous chronic diseases.

Low carb eating offers a range of health benefits, from weight loss and improved metabolic health to enhanced mental clarity and a reduced risk of chronic disease. By focusing on a diverse intake of nutrient-dense, low carb foods, beginners can embark on a dietary journey that not only promotes immediate health improvements but also lays the foundation for long-term wellness and disease prevention.

How to Transition to a Low Carb Lifestyle

Transitioning to a low carb lifestyle is a journey that begins with understanding the essence of what it means to reduce carbohydrate intake and embrace foods that fuel your body more efficiently. , this shift is not merely about eliminating certain foods but about reimagining your diet to prioritize health and vitality. A low carb diet focuses on reducing sugars and starches, replacing them with vegetables, healthy fats, and proteins to encourage the body to burn fat for energy.

The first step in this transformation involves education and preparation. Learning about the types of foods that fit within a low carb framework is crucial. A comprehensive food list serves as the cornerstone of this education, outlining which foods to enjoy freely, such as leafy greens, non-starchy vegetables, meats, fish, eggs, nuts, and seeds, along with specific dairy products like cheese and Greek yogurt. Equally important is understanding which foods to limit or avoid, including sugary sweets, grains, high carb fruits, and processed foods.

Preparation extends beyond knowledge; it's about setting up your environment for success. This means reorganizing your kitchen, pantry, and fridge to remove high-carb temptations and stocking up on low carb essentials. This process not only makes it easier to stick to your new diet but also helps in mentally committing to the change.

Gradual changes often yield more sustainable results. Rather than an abrupt overhaul, start by reducing sugar and refined carbs, incorporating more vegetables and proteins into your meals. This slower approach helps your body and taste preferences adjust without the shock of a sudden dietary change, making the transition smoother and more manageable.

Meal planning becomes an invaluable tool in maintaining a low carb lifestyle. Planning your meals and snacks ahead of time ensures that you have the right foods on hand when hunger strikes, preventing fallbacks into old, carb-heavy eating habits. It also introduces variety and creativity into your diet, making the lifestyle enjoyable and sustainable.

Understanding how to read and interpret food labels is another essential skill. It enables you to make informed choices about what to include in your diet, especially when it comes to hidden sugars and carbs in packaged foods. This vigilance ensures you stay within your carb limits while exploring new foods that fit your low carb criteria.

Physical activity, while not directly related to your diet, complements the low carb lifestyle by improving metabolism and enhancing the benefits of your dietary changes. Incorporating regular exercise into your routine can accelerate weight loss, improve insulin sensitivity, and boost your overall sense of well-being.

Support from a community or network of individuals who are also embracing a low carb lifestyle can significantly enhance your journey. Sharing experiences, challenges, and successes provides motivation, encouragement, and valuable insights that can help navigate the transition more effectively.

Finally, patience and self-compassion are key. Transitioning to a low carb lifestyle is a significant change that requires time to adjust, both physically and mentally. Setbacks are part of the journey, but with persistence and a positive mindset, adapting to a low carb lifestyle becomes not just a possibility but a rewarding and sustainable way of life.

By embracing these strategies and integrating them into your daily routine, the transition to a low carb lifestyle becomes a journey of discovery, health, and fulfillment, guided by the foundational principles outlined in a beginner's low carb diet food list.

Understanding Macronutrients

When embarking on a low carb diet, a fundamental step is to grasp the concept of macronutrients—carbohydrates, proteins, and fats. These are the primary components of every diet, and understanding their roles is crucial for anyone looking to follow a low carb lifestyle effectively.

Carbohydrates, often the main focus in low carb diets, are typically reduced to promote weight loss and improve metabolic health. This group includes sugars, starches, and fibers found in fruits, vegetables, grains, and dairy products. On a low carb diet, the emphasis is on minimizing sugar and starch intake while focusing on high-fiber foods such as leafy greens and non-starchy vegetables. This shift helps stabilize blood sugar levels, reduce insulin spikes, and encourage the body to burn fat for energy instead of relying on carbohydrates.

Proteins are essential for the repair and growth of tissues, and they play a vital role in immune function, hormone production, and other bodily processes. In a low carb diet, protein sources such as meat, poultry, fish, and plant-based alternatives become a significant part of meals. However, it's important to balance protein intake to prevent excessive consumption, which can lead to kidney strain in susceptible individuals and potentially interrupt ketosis, a state where the body burns fat as its primary source of fuel.

Fats, once vilified, are now recognized for their essential roles in a healthy diet, especially in low carb eating plans. Healthy fats from sources like avocados, nuts, seeds, olive oil, and fatty fish are encouraged. These fats provide energy, support cell growth, protect organs, and help absorb vitamins. They also contribute to satiety, making it easier to stick to a low carb diet by reducing overall hunger.

Understanding the impact of each macronutrient on the body helps beginners make informed food choices. For instance, replacing high carb foods with those rich in healthy fats and moderate in proteins can shift the body's metabolism from carb-burning to fat-burning, a principle at the heart of the low carb diet. Moreover, understanding macronutrients aids in creating a balanced diet that supports long-term health and wellness beyond just weight loss.

In relation to a low carb diet, this knowledge empowers individuals to tailor their diet to their personal health goals, activity levels, and metabolic health. By focusing on the quality and balance of macronutrients, beginners can navigate the low carb lifestyle with confidence, ensuring they not only lose weight but also nurture their body's overall health. This approach supports a sustainable transition to healthier eating habits, highlighting the importance of informed food choices in achieving lasting dietary success.

Preparing for Your Low Carb Journey

Setting Realistic Goals

Setting realistic goals is a critical first step for anyone embarking on a low carb journey, especially who are navigating through the myriad of food choices and dietary adjustments. It lays the foundation for a sustainable lifestyle change, ensuring that the transition to low carb eating is not only effective but also achievable and rewarding.

The essence of setting realistic goals in the context of a low carb diet involves aligning expectations with individual lifestyle, health status, and personal preferences. It's about creating a vision for one's health that is both aspirational and grounded in reality. This process starts with understanding one's current eating habits and nutritional knowledge and then gradually introducing changes that are both significant and manageable.

Begin by assessing your current diet and identify the carb-heavy foods that are staples in your meals. Recognizing these will help you understand the adjustments needed to transition to a low carb diet.

For many, this might mean reducing or eliminating bread, pasta, sugary snacks, and other processed foods high in carbohydrates.

Next, establish clear, measurable goals. Instead of setting a vague goal like "eat less sugar," specify how much sugar you will cut from your diet and by when. For example, "reduce added sugar intake to less than 25 grams per day within the next month." This specificity makes your goal more tangible and provides a clear benchmark for success.

It's also important to set both short-term and long-term goals. Short-term goals might include learning to read nutritional labels to identify carb content, while a long-term goal could be achieving and maintaining a healthy weight or improving your blood sugar levels if you have diabetes.

When setting goals, consider the SMART criteria—Specific, Measurable, Achievable, Relevant, and Time-bound. This framework ensures that your goals are well-defined and within reach. For instance, a SMART goal for a beginner might be, "I will replace two servings of starchy vegetables with low carb alternatives like leafy greens or cruciferous vegetables at least five days a week for the next month."

Acknowledge the importance of flexibility in your goal-setting. Life happens, and there will be moments when adhering strictly to your low carb diet might be challenging. Be prepared to adjust your goals as needed, whether it's due to changes in your schedule, unexpected events, or simply discovering what works best for your body.

Moreover, consider the psychological aspects of goal-setting. Motivation can fluctuate, and it's essential to prepare for moments of temptation or setbacks. Create a support system, whether it's friends, family, or online communities, who understand your goals and can offer encouragement. Celebrate your successes, no matter how small, to keep motivation high.

In conclusion, setting realistic goals is about more than just deciding to eat fewer carbs. It's a comprehensive approach that involves understanding your current habits, creating specific and achievable objectives, preparing for challenges, and celebrating progress. By taking the time to set thoughtful, realistic goals, beginners can navigate their low carb journey with confidence, making lasting changes that go beyond temporary dieting to foster a healthier, more vibrant lifestyle.

Cleaning Out Your Pantry

Embarking on a low carb journey often starts with a simple yet transformative step: cleaning out your pantry. This initial act is not just about removing temptation; it's about setting the stage for a new, healthier lifestyle. As beginners transition to a low carb diet, the pantry becomes a reflection of their new eating philosophy—out with the old, high-carb staples and in with the new, low carb essentials.

The process begins with identifying and removing foods high in carbohydrates. These typically include items like pasta, white rice, bread, cereal, and baked goods. Sugary snacks, sodas, and other sweetened beverages also fall into this category. It might be challenging to part with these familiar items, but recognizing their limited place in a low carb diet is crucial for long-term success.

Next, focus on high-carb condiments and canned goods that can sabotage low carb efforts. Many sauces, dressings, and spreads are laden with added sugars and unhealthy fats. Canned fruits and vegetables, often preserved in syrup or added sugars, should also be replaced with their fresh or frozen counterparts, which are more nutrient-dense and lower in carbs.

After clearing out the high-carb foods, the next step is to restock with low carb alternatives. This includes a variety of non-starchy vegetables, such as leafy greens, broccoli, cauliflower, and zucchini, which will become dietary staples. For those who enjoy baking or cooking, almond flour and coconut flour are excellent low carb substitutes for traditional wheat flour.

Quality proteins are also essential. Stock up on canned or pouched proteins like tuna, salmon, and chicken for quick, easy meals. Nuts and seeds, along with their butters, offer healthy fats and are perfect for snacking or adding to recipes.

Healthy fats are crucial on a low carb diet, so olive oil, coconut oil, and avocado oil should have a prominent place in your pantry. These fats are not only cooking essentials but also key to feeling satiated and energized.

For flavoring, a variety of spices and herbs can enhance meals without adding carbs. Stocking up on these allows for creativity in cooking and helps keep meals interesting and flavorful. Additionally, consider low-carb sweeteners like stevia or erythritol for those occasional sweet treats without the carb load.

One overlooked aspect of pantry cleaning is organization. A well-organized pantry makes it easier to maintain your low carb lifestyle.

Group items together by category, and make your low carb essentials easily accessible. This not only helps with meal planning and preparation but also reinforces your new dietary habits each time you open the pantry door.

Finally, consider your pantry clean-out as an ongoing process rather than a one-time event. As you progress in your low carb journey, you'll discover new favorites and perhaps realize that some items no longer fit your dietary goals. Periodically reassessing the contents of your pantry ensures that your food choices continue to align with your health objectives.

Cleaning out your pantry is a vital first step in preparing for your low carb journey. It symbolizes your commitment to change and lays the foundation for a healthier lifestyle. By removing high-carb foods and stocking up on low carb essentials, you're setting yourself up for success, making it easier to adhere to your new diet and achieve your health goals.

Kitchen Essentials for Low Carb Cooking

Embarking on a low carb journey involves more than just stocking your pantry with the right foods. It also means having the right tools in your kitchen to make preparing delicious, low-carb meals as easy and efficient as possible. Here's a comprehensive guide to the kitchen essentials that will support your low carb cooking adventures, ensuring you have everything you need to whip up healthy, satisfying meals.

- **Quality Knives**: A sharp chef's knife and a paring knife are indispensable for efficiently prepping vegetables, meats, and other fresh ingredients that form the basis of a low carb diet. Investing in quality knives makes chopping and slicing quicker and safer, encouraging you to use a variety of fresh produce in your cooking.

- **Cutting Boards**: Having multiple cutting boards allows you to prevent cross-contamination between raw meats and vegetables. Opt for boards made of bamboo or hardwood, as they are durable and less likely to harbor bacteria.

- **Non-Stick Skillet**: A good non-stick skillet is essential for cooking everything from omelets and frittatas to sautéed vegetables and seared meats. It reduces the need for added fats and oils, keeping your meals as healthy as possible.

- **Food Processor**: This versatile tool is a time-saver for chopping vegetables, grinding nuts and seeds, making cauliflower rice, or preparing homemade nut butters. A food processor makes it easier to incorporate a variety of textures and flavors into your low carb meals.

- **Spiralizer**: A spiralizer turns vegetables like zucchini, carrots, and squash into "noodles," offering a low carb alternative to traditional pasta. It's a fun way to add vegetables to your diet and experiment with different recipes.

- **Measuring Cups and Spoons**: Precise measurements are crucial in low carb cooking, especially when baking. Measuring cups and spoons help you ensure that you're sticking to your carb limits while preparing recipes.

- **Slow Cooker or Instant Pot**: These appliances are excellent for busy individuals. They allow for easy, set-it-and-forget-it meals, such as stews, soups, and tender meats, that can be prepared with minimal effort but deliver maximum flavor.

- **Blender:** A high-powered blender is useful for making smoothies, pureed soups, and low carb sauces. It can also be used to blend nuts and seeds into flours or milk, offering alternatives to traditional high carb options.

- **Baking Sheets and Silicone Mats**: For roasting vegetables or making homemade low carb snacks, baking sheets paired with silicone baking mats are essential. They provide a non-stick surface, reducing the need for extra oils, and ensure even cooking.

- **Glass Storage Containers**: Proper storage is key to maintaining the freshness of your prepared meals and ingredients. Glass containers are preferable as they don't hold onto odors or stains and are generally safer for reheating food than plastic containers.

- **Spice Grinder**: Freshly ground spices enhance the flavor of any dish without adding carbs. A small spice grinder can be used for spices, allowing you to explore a range of flavors in your cooking.

Having the right tools at your disposal can significantly impact your success and enjoyment of a low carb lifestyle. These kitchen essentials not only help in preparing a wide variety of low carb meals but also ensure that cooking and meal prep become a pleasurable and integral part of your health journey. As you become more accustomed to low carb cooking, you might find certain tools become indispensable, reflecting your unique approach to food and wellness.

Reading Food Labels for Carb Content

Reading food labels is a critical skill for anyone embarking on a low carb journey. This practice helps you understand what's in the foods you eat and allows you to make informed decisions aligned with your dietary goals. , deciphering these labels might seem daunting at first, but with a bit of guidance, it becomes an invaluable tool in maintaining a low carb lifestyle.

The first step in reading food labels for carb content is to look at the serving size. This figure is crucial because all the nutritional information listed pertains to this specific amount of food. Misjudging the serving size can lead to unintentional overconsumption of carbs.

Next, direct your attention to the total carbohydrates listed on the label. This number encompasses all types of carbohydrates in the food, including dietary fibers, sugars, and other starches. Since low carb diets focus on reducing sugar and starch intake while encouraging fiber, understanding this breakdown is essential.

Dietary fiber is listed under the total carbohydrates and can be subtracted from the total carbs when calculating your intake. This is because fiber, while technically a carbohydrate, is not digested and absorbed by the body in the same way other carbs are. It doesn't raise blood sugar levels, making high-fiber foods excellent choices for a low carb diet.

Sugars, also listed under carbohydrates, require careful consideration. This includes both added sugars and naturally occurring sugars found in foods. For a low carb diet, it's crucial to minimize added sugars as much as possible. Foods high in added sugars provide empty calories and can quickly exceed daily carb limits.

Many food labels now differentiate between total sugars and added sugars, making it easier to identify foods that fit into a low carb diet. Opting for foods with low or no added sugars can help keep your carb intake in check.

Another aspect to be aware of is sugar alcohols, which are often found in low carb or sugar-free products. While they have a lower impact on blood sugar levels than regular sugar, their effect can vary, and some people may need to count them as part of their total carb intake.

Understanding the nuances of food labels allows beginners to navigate the complexities of managing carb intake more effectively. By focusing on the net carb content (total carbohydrates minus dietary fiber and, sometimes, sugar alcohols) instead of just the total carbs, you can make choices that align better with a low carb diet.

In addition to carbs, it's beneficial to pay attention to the protein and fat content. A balanced low carb diet also involves adequate protein intake and healthy fats, which can contribute to satiety and overall nutritional balance.

Incorporating this practice into your shopping routine can significantly impact your success on a low carb diet. It not only helps in making better food choices but also in understanding how different foods affect your body's carb tolerance and overall health. As you become more accustomed to reading food labels for carb content, you'll likely find it easier to stay within your daily carb limits, ensuring a smoother transition to and maintenance of a low carb lifestyle.

Comprehensive Low Carb Food List

Vegetables: From Leafy Greens to Cruciferous Veggies

Vegetables are not only low in carbs but are also rich in essential nutrients like vitamins, minerals, and fiber. Here, we'll explore a selection of vegetables from leafy greens to cruciferous veggies, highlighting their carb counts and nutritional benefits in a tabular format for easy reference.

Vegetable Type	Examples	Net Carbs (per 100g)	Usefulness
Leafy Greens	Spinach, Kale, Swiss Chard	1-3g	High in vitamins A, C, K, and minerals like iron and calcium. Great for salads and smoothies.
Cruciferous Vegetables	Broccoli, Cauliflower, Brussels	2-5g	Rich in fiber and vitamin C. They have cancer-fighting properties and

Vegetable Type	Examples	Net Carbs (per 100g)	Usefulness
	Sprouts		can be roasted or steamed.
Salad Vegetables	Lettuce, Cucumber, Radishes	1-3g	Contain high water content and essential nutrients with minimal carbs. Ideal for fresh salads.
Stem Vegetables	Asparagus, Celery	2-3g	Good sources of vitamins A, C, K, and folate. Suitable for steaming, grilling, or as snack sticks.
Alliums	Garlic, Onions	5-9g	Provide flavor depth to dishes. They have anti-inflammatory and antioxidant properties.
Nightshades	Bell Peppers, Eggplant	3-6g	High in vitamins C and K, potassium, and fiber. Versatile for grilling, baking, or in stir-fries.

Vegetable Type	Examples	Net Carbs (per 100g)	Usefulness
Squashes	Zucchini, Pumpkin	2-7g	Rich in vitamins A and C, and low in carbs. Perfect for baking, soups, or spiralized as 'zoodles'.
Root Vegetables	Radishes, Turnips	2-4g	Lower in carbs than other root veggies. They provide a crunchy texture and are rich in fiber.

Leafy greens and cruciferous vegetables are particularly beneficial for their low carb content and high nutritional density, making them staples in any low carb diet. Salad vegetables like lettuce and cucumber are perfect for adding volume and freshness to meals without significantly increasing carb intake.

Stem vegetables and alliums, although slightly higher in carbs, offer unique flavors and health benefits that can enhance the quality of a low carb diet. Nightshades and squashes provide versatility in cooking methods, from grilling to baking, allowing for creative low carb dishes. Lastly, select root vegetables like radishes and turnips can be included in moderation, offering fiber and nutrients while keeping carb counts in check.

Proteins: Meat, Poultry, Fish, and Plant-Based Options

Each entry includes the protein source, its low carb count, and its usefulness in a low carb diet, providing a comprehensive overview for anyone following or considering such a lifestyle.

Protein Source	Low Carb Count (per 100g)	Usefulness
Meat		
Beef (lean cuts)	0g	High in protein and iron, beef is a staple in low carb diets for muscle repair and energy.
Pork (lean cuts)	0g	Provides high-quality protein and essential vitamins like B6 and B12.
Lamb	0g	Rich in protein and important nutrients like iron, zinc, and vitamin B12.

Protein Source	Low Carb Count (per 100g)	Usefulness
Poultry		
Chicken Breast	0g	Lean source of protein that helps with muscle maintenance and repair.
Turkey (skinless)	0g	Another lean protein, turkey is also rich in selenium and vitamins B3 and B6.
Duck	0g	Higher in fat, providing a good source of protein and a richer flavor.
Fish		
Salmon	0g	Offers omega-3 fatty acids for heart health and is a great protein

Protein Source	Low Carb Count (per 100g)	Usefulness
		source.
Tuna (fresh or canned in water)	0g	High in protein and omega-3s, convenient for quick meals.
Cod	0g	Low in fat and high in protein, making it a great choice for weight management.
Plant-Based Options		
Tofu	1-2g	Versatile protein source that's also a good source of iron and calcium.
Tempeh	9g	Fermented, making it easier to digest, and rich in protein and fiber.
Seitan	5g	High in protein, making it a popular

Protein Source	Low Carb Count (per 100g)	Usefulness
		meat substitute, though it's derived from wheat gluten.
Almonds	22g (carbs)	While higher in carbs, they're a good source of protein and healthy fats.
Chia Seeds	42g (carbs)	High in fiber, which can offset the carb count, and rich in protein and omega-3s.

It's important to consider the overall carb limit and dietary needs when choosing protein sources, especially for those opting for plant-based options, as some may have higher carb counts due to their fiber content. Including a wide range of proteins can help ensure nutritional balance, offering essential vitamins, minerals, and fatty acids vital for health and wellbeing on a low carb diet.

Fats: Healthy Oils, Nuts, and Seeds

Fats play a crucial role in nutrition, providing energy, supporting cell growth, and assisting in the absorption of certain vitamins. They are also key for satiety and flavor in a low carb lifestyle. Below is a detailed table showcasing various healthy fats, their low carb count, and their usefulness in a low carb diet.

Food Category	Specific Food	Net Carbs (per 100g/serving)	Usefulness in a Low Carb Diet
Healthy Oils	Olive oil	0g	High in monounsaturated fats; beneficial for heart health; great for salads and low-heat cooking.
	Coconut oil	0g	Contains medium-chain triglycerides (MCTs); supports ketosis; ideal for cooking at high temperatures.
	Avocado oil	0g	Rich in monounsaturated fats; high smoke point makes it versatile for cooking and dressing.

Food Category	Specific Food	Net Carbs (per 100g/serving)	Usefulness in a Low Carb Diet
	MCT oil	0g	Direct source of MCTs; supports energy levels and ketosis; popular in keto coffee and smoothies.
Nuts	Almonds	22g (net 9g)	High in vitamin E and magnesium; provides sustained energy; great for snacking or as a salad topping.
	Pecans	14g (net 4g)	Low in carbs, high in dietary fiber; rich in antioxidants; perfect for snacking or homemade low carb desserts.
	Macadamia nuts	14g (net 5g)	Highest in monounsaturated fats; low in carbs; ideal for a keto diet for satiety and flavor.
	Walnuts	14g (net 2g)	Rich in omega-3 fatty

Food Category	Specific Food	Net Carbs (per 100g/serving)	Usefulness in a Low Carb Diet
			acids; supports brain health; good for snacking or adding to low carb dishes.
Seeds	Chia seeds	42g (net 8g)	High in fiber and omega-3s; can absorb water to form a gel, useful for low carb puddings and smoothies.
	Flaxseeds	29g (net 1.6g)	Rich in fiber, lignans, and omega-3 fatty acids; useful for adding to low carb breads or as a meal topping.
	Pumpkin seeds	54g (net 5g)	High in magnesium, iron, and zinc; adds crunch and nutrients to salads or as a standalone snack.
	Sunflower seeds	20g (net 6g)	Good source of vitamin E and selenium; versatile for snacking or

Food Category	Specific Food	Net Carbs (per 100g/serving)	Usefulness in a Low Carb Diet
			enhancing low carb dishes.

Oils provide a pure fat source with minimal to no carbs, making them ideal for maintaining ketosis and ensuring adequate fat intake. Nuts and seeds, while containing some net carbs, offer a good mix of fiber, healthy fats, and other vital nutrients, contributing to a balanced, nutritious low carb diet. They can be easily incorporated into meals and snacks to add texture, flavor, and nutritional value, supporting overall health and dietary satisfaction.

Dairy: Choosing Low Carb Options

For individuals following a low carb lifestyle, navigating the dairy aisle can be a bit tricky. Dairy products not only play a vital role in providing essential nutrients like calcium, vitamin D, and protein but also add richness and flavor to low carb meals.

However, not all dairy products are created equal when it comes to carb content. Here's a detailed table to guide you through choosing low carb options, highlighting their carb count and usefulness:

Dairy Product	Carb Count (per 100g)	Usefulness
Heavy Cream	2.8g	Adds creaminess to coffee or recipes without a high carb load.
Greek Yogurt (Plain, Full-Fat)	4g	High in protein and probiotics; good for breakfast or snacks.
Cheese (Hard Varieties)	1.3g	Versatile, high in protein and fat, suitable for snacks or adding flavor to dishes.
Butter	0.1g	Provides healthy fats, great for cooking and adding flavor.

Dairy Product	Carb Count (per 100g)	Usefulness
Cottage Cheese (Full-Fat)	3.4g	Good source of protein; can be eaten as a snack or added to meals.
Sour Cream (Full-Fat)	2.9g	Can be used in recipes to add creaminess with minimal carbs.
Cream Cheese (Full-Fat)	4.1g	Useful in baking, sauces, or as a spread, while keeping carbs low.

Notes on the Table:

- **Carb Count**: The carbohydrate content can vary slightly between brands and specific products, so always check the label. The counts provided here are average values.

- **Heavy Cream**: With its high fat content and low carb count, heavy cream is excellent for enriching coffee or making low carb desserts and sauces.

- **Greek Yogurt**: Opt for plain, full-fat versions to minimize added sugars. Greek yogurt is perfect for a quick breakfast or a satisfying snack, providing probiotics and protein.

- **Cheese**: Hard varieties like cheddar, parmesan, and swiss have lower carb counts compared to softer cheeses. Cheese is incredibly versatile, serving as a delicious snack on its own or as a flavorful addition to recipes.

- **Butter**: Almost carb-free, butter is excellent for frying, baking, or simply as a topping, adding quality fats to your diet.

- **Cottage Cheese**: Choosing full-fat versions ensures lower carb content. Cottage cheese works well in both sweet and savory contexts, from toppings to standalone snacks.

- **Sour Cream**: Ideal for adding tanginess to recipes without significantly increasing the carb count. It pairs well with low carb vegetables and in dips.

- **Cream Cheese**: Full-fat cream cheese is a staple in low carb baking, offering texture and flavor with relatively low carbs.

When incorporating dairy into a low carb diet, it's essential to opt for full-fat versions where possible. These not only have lower carb counts but also provide essential fats that can help keep you full and satisfied, making it easier to stick to your low carb goals. Additionally, always read labels carefully, as some products may contain added sugars or fillers that increase the carb content.

Fruits: Berries and Other Low Carb Choices

Certain fruits, particularly berries and some other specific options, fit well within the parameters of low carb eating plans due to their lower net carb content and nutritional benefits. Here's a table highlighting some of these fruits, including berries and other low carb choices, their approximate net carb counts per standard serving size, and their health benefits, which make them valuable additions to a low carb diet.

Fruit Type	Serving Size	Net Carbs (g)	Health Benefits
Berries			
Strawberries	1 cup (sliced)	9	High in vitamin C and antioxidants, supports immune function and skin health.
Raspberries	1 cup	7	Rich in fiber, vitamins, and minerals; may help improve digestive health.
Blackberries	1 cup	6	High in vitamins C and K, fiber, and antioxidants; supports heart health.

Fruit Type	Serving Size	Net Carbs (g)	Health Benefits
Blueberries	1 cup	17	Packed with antioxidants and vitamin C; supports brain health and heart function.
Other Fruits			
Avocado	1 whole (medium)	3	Rich in healthy fats, fiber, and potassium; supports heart health and can help improve cholesterol.
Coconut	1 cup (shredded)	5	High in fiber and MCTs (Medium Chain Triglycerides); supports metabolism and brain health.
Olives	1 cup (sliced)	4	High in vitamin E and healthy fats; anti-inflammatory and antioxidant properties.
Tomatoes	1 cup (chopped)	4	Contains lycopene, vitamins C and K; supports heart health and provides antioxidant benefits.
Lemons/Limes	1 whole (medium)	4	High in vitamin C; supports immune function and can aid digestion.
Rhubarb	1 cup	3	High in fiber, vitamin K, and

Fruit Type	Serving Size	Net Carbs (g)	Health Benefits
	(diced)		calcium; supports bone health.
Cantaloupe	1 cup (cubed)	11	Rich in vitamins A and C; supports immune system and skin health.

Berries stand out as an excellent option due to their low net carb content and high nutrient density, including antioxidants, which can combat oxidative stress and inflammation. Avocado, although not typically considered fruit in culinary contexts, is a powerhouse of healthy fats and fiber, making it a staple in low carb diets. Other fruits like olives and tomatoes offer healthy fats and essential nutrients, including antioxidants, without significantly increasing carb intake.

Understanding the carb content and health benefits of these fruits enables individuals following a low carb diet to make informed choices, ensuring they can enjoy the sweetness and nutritional benefits of fruit without compromising their dietary goals. Integrating these fruits into a low carb diet can enhance dietary variety, contribute to overall nutrient intake, and support health and well-being.

Beverages: What to Drink on a Low Carb Diet

When following a low carb diet, it's not just the food that counts—beverages play a significant role in your daily carb intake and can either support or hinder your progress. Below is a comprehensive guide on what beverages to include in your low carb diet, focusing on their carb count and usefulness to your health and diet goals.

Beverage Type	Low Carb Count (per serving)	Usefulness
Water	0g	Essential for hydration, metabolism, and overall health. Can be infused with lemon or mint for flavor.
Sparkling Water	0g	A refreshing alternative to still water, with no carbs. Helps satisfy the desire for carbonated drinks.
Black Coffee	0g	Contains antioxidants and can boost metabolism. Drink it black or with a splash of heavy cream to keep it low carb.

Beverage Type	Low Carb Count (per serving)	Usefulness
Tea (Black, Green, Herbal)	0g	Offers a variety of antioxidants. Herbal teas can provide calming effects or digestive aid without adding carbs.
Bone Broth	0-2g	Nutrient-rich, supports gut health, and provides essential minerals and amino acids.
Unsweetened Almond Milk	1-2g	A low carb, plant-based milk alternative rich in vitamin E and great for coffee, tea, or smoothies.
Coconut Water	9-12g (per 8 ounces)	Although higher in carbs, it's a good source of potassium and magnesium. Best consumed in moderation.
Vegetable Juice	5-10g (per 8 ounces)	Choose low-carb vegetables like tomatoes or cucumbers. Avoid store-bought versions that may contain added sugars.
Diet Soda	0g	While carb-free, it's best consumed in moderation due to the presence of artificial sweeteners.

Beverage Type	Low Carb Count (per serving)	Usefulness
Dry Wine	2-4g (per 5 ounces)	Low in carbs, but alcohol consumption should be moderated. Red wine has beneficial antioxidants.
Light Beer	2-6g (per 12 ounces)	Some light beers offer lower carb content for those who prefer beer. Consume in moderation.
Hard Liquor	0g	Spirits like vodka, whiskey, gin, and rum have no carbs but should be consumed straight or with a no-carb mixer.

This table serves as a guide to making beverage choices on a low carb diet. Hydration is key, and water should be your primary drink. When you want something different, black coffee and a variety of teas are excellent options, offering health benefits along with hydration without compromising your carb limit.

For those who miss milk, unsweetened almond milk presents a fantastic low carb alternative, perfect for smoothies or coffee. If you're looking for electrolytes after a workout, coconut water can be a good option, though it's higher in carbs and should be consumed in moderation.

Vegetable juices can be nutritious but watch out for the carb content and make sure they are made from low-carb veggies and without added sugars. Diet sodas and alcohol can fit into a low carb diet but remember to enjoy these in moderation due to their potential impact on cravings, blood sugar levels, and overall health.

Choosing the right beverages is crucial for staying within your daily carb limit and ensuring your low carb diet is as effective and enjoyable as possible. With careful selection, you can enjoy a variety of drinks that contribute to your hydration and dietary goals without compromising on taste or variety.

Herbs and Spices: Flavoring Your Food the Low Carb Way

When transitioning to a low carb lifestyle, one might worry about the potential monotony of flavor in their diet. However, the use of herbs and spices not only adds zest and depth to your meals but also comes with minimal to no carb content, making them perfect for flavoring food the low carb way.

Below is a detailed table that includes a selection of herbs and spices, their carb count, and their usefulness in a low carb diet. This guide will help beginners incorporate a variety of flavors into their meals without compromising their carb limits.

Herb/Spice	Carb Count (per 1 tsp)	Usefulness in Low Carb Diet
Basil	0.1g	Fresh or dried, basil adds a sweet, herbal freshness to salads, sauces, and meats. It's particularly popular in Italian and Southeast Asian cuisines.
Cinnamon	0.8g	With its warm, sweet flavor, cinnamon is ideal for adding depth

Herb/Spice	Carb Count (per 1 tsp)	Usefulness in Low Carb Diet
		to desserts and beverages. It can also enhance the natural sweetness of low carb fruits like berries.
Cumin	0.9g	This earthy, aromatic spice is a staple in Indian, Middle Eastern, and Mexican cuisines. It's perfect for seasoning meat, vegetables, and soups.
Garlic Powder	2g	Offering a concentrated burst of flavor, garlic powder is a convenient way to add a kick to meats, vegetables, and sauces.
Oregano	0.4g	With its strong, slightly bitter flavor, oregano is great for enhancing the taste of Italian and Greek dishes.
Paprika	0.6g	This sweet or smoky spice adds vibrant color and flavor to chicken, fish, and vegetable dishes.
Rosemary	0.2g	Rosemary's pine-like aroma and flavor complement a wide range of dishes, from roasted meats to

Herb/Spice	Carb Count (per 1 tsp)	Usefulness in Low Carb Diet
		focaccia.
Thyme	0.8g	With its subtle, dry aroma and slightly minty flavor, thyme is versatile in seasoning chicken, soups, and vegetables.
Turmeric	0.9g	Known for its anti-inflammatory properties, turmeric adds a warm, bitter flavor and vibrant color to curries and rice dishes.
Chili Powder	0.8g	A blend of ground chilis and other spices, chili powder adds heat and complexity to Tex-Mex and Indian dishes.
Ginger	0.9g	Fresh or dried, ginger adds a spicy, warm flavor to dishes and drinks. It's particularly good in Asian recipes and tea.
Parsley	0.1g	Fresh parsley has a clean, slightly peppery taste that brightens up savory dishes and garnishes.
Saffron	0.7g	The world's most expensive spice,

Herb/Spice	Carb Count (per 1 tsp)	Usefulness in Low Carb Diet
		saffron adds a rich gold color and a distinctive taste to Mediterranean dishes.
Cayenne Pepper	0.6g	This hot spice adds significant heat and a touch of sweetness to dishes, perfect for those looking to spice up their meals.

Incorporating herbs and spices into your low carb diet is not only beneficial for enhancing flavor without adding carbs but also for their health benefits. Many herbs and spices contain antioxidants and have anti-inflammatory properties, supporting overall wellness. As seen in the table, the carb counts are minimal, often less than 1 gram per teaspoon, making them an excellent option for adding variety and depth to your low carb meals. This approach allows beginners and seasoned low carb dieters alike to enjoy a diverse and flavorful diet without compromising their nutritional goals.

Foods to Avoid on a Low Carb Diet

High Carb Vegetables and Legumes

High Carb Vegetables and Legumes	Average Carbohydrates (per 100g serving)	Why to Avoid in a Low Carb Diet
Potatoes	17g	Potatoes are rich in starch, a type of carbohydrate that can quickly raise blood sugar levels. In a low carb diet, minimizing foods that spike blood sugar is key to maintaining ketosis, a state where the body burns fat for energy.
Sweet potatoes	20g	Similar to regular potatoes, sweet potatoes are high in carbs and can disrupt the metabolic state desired in low carb diets. While they are a source of vitamins and minerals, their high starch content makes them less ideal for

High Carb Vegetables and Legumes	Average Carbohydrates (per serving)	100g	Why to Avoid in a Low Carb Diet
			strict low carb intake.
Corn	19g		Corn is another vegetable that's high in carbohydrates, primarily in the form of sugars and starch. It can contribute to higher blood sugar levels, making it unsuitable for a low carb diet focused on fat burning and stable insulin levels.
Peas	14g		Peas contain a moderate amount of carbohydrates, including natural sugars and starch. For those strictly monitoring their carb intake, peas may be consumed in very small quantities or avoided to stay within low carb guidelines.

High Carb Vegetables and Legumes	Average Carbohydrates (per 100g serving)	Why to Avoid in a Low Carb Diet
Butternut squash	12g	While butternut squash is packed with nutrients, its carb content is relatively high for a vegetable, consisting mainly of sugars and starch. In a low carb diet, consuming it may require careful portion control.
Parsnips	18g	Parsnips are root vegetables that are high in sugars and starch. Their high carbohydrate content can interfere with ketosis or other low carb diet goals, making them less favorable for inclusion.
Beans (Black, Pinto, Kidney)	20-25g	Beans are legumes that are high in protein but also come with a significant amount of carbohydrates. Although they are rich in fiber, their net carb content may still be too high for a strict low carb diet.

High Carb Vegetables and Legumes	Average Carbohydrates (per 100g serving)	Why to Avoid in a Low Carb Diet
Lentils	20g	Lentils are another legume that, despite their health benefits, including high protein and fiber, also contain a substantial amount of carbs. Their inclusion in a low carb diet requires careful management of serving sizes.

While these vegetables and legumes provide nutritional benefits, such as vitamins, minerals, and fiber, their high carbohydrate content makes them less ideal for those following a strict low carb diet. In a low carb lifestyle, the goal is to minimize carb intake to encourage the body to use fat as its primary energy source. Consuming high carb vegetables and legumes can disrupt this process, leading to potential spikes in blood sugar and making it more challenging to maintain a state of ketosis or manage insulin sensitivity.

However, it's worth noting that "low carb" does not mean "no carb," and individual tolerance levels can vary. Some people following a more liberal low carb diet may be able to include small portions of these higher carb foods without negative effects. The key is to understand your body's response and adjust your diet accordingly, prioritizing vegetables and legumes that align with your carb intake goals.

Sugary Foods and Drinks

Sugary Foods and Drinks	Reasons to Avoid	Low Carb Alternatives
Soft Drinks & Energy Drinks	High in added sugars and empty calories, contributing to blood sugar spikes, weight gain, and an increased risk of type 2 diabetes.	Sparkling water with a splash of natural fruit flavor, herbal teas, or black coffee.
Candy & Chocolate Bars (traditional)	Loaded with sugars and fats that can lead to rapid increases in blood glucose levels and contribute to dental problems and obesity.	Dark chocolate (over 70% cocoa) in moderation or sugar-free candies made with stevia or erythritol.
Baked Goods (Cookies, Cakes, Pastries)	Often contain high amounts of sugar and refined flours, which are quickly converted into glucose in the body, spiking insulin levels.	Baked goods made with almond flour, coconut flour, or other low carb flours and sweetened with low glycemic index sweeteners.

Sugary Foods and Drinks	Reasons to Avoid	Low Carb Alternatives
Ice Cream	Traditional ice cream is high in sugar and fat, contributing to weight gain and disrupting insulin sensitivity.	Low carb ice cream made with keto-friendly sweeteners or frozen berries blended with heavy cream for a homemade alternative.
Fruit Juices	Even 100% fruit juice can contain as much sugar as a soda, lacking the fiber of whole fruits, leading to quicker absorption of sugar.	Water infused with fresh fruit slices or vegetable juices with no added sugars, focusing on leafy greens.
Sports Drinks	Marketed as health beverages but often contain high levels of sugars and artificial flavorings, providing more energy than the average person needs.	Electrolyte-infused water without added sugars or homemade electrolyte drinks using lemon juice, salt, and a sweetener like stevia.
Processed Fruit Snacks	Can be misleadingly marketed as healthy but	Whole fruits, especially those low in carbs like

Sugary Foods and Drinks	Reasons to Avoid	Low Carb Alternatives
	are usually high in added sugars and contain little to no real fruit.	berries, or homemade fruit snacks made with pureed fruit and gelatin.
Flavored Yogurts	Often low in fat but high in added sugars, which can negate the benefits of the live cultures present in yogurt.	Plain Greek yogurt sweetened with a bit of stevia or mixed with low carb fruits like raspberries or blackberries.
Granola Bars	Perceived as a healthy snack but frequently loaded with sugars and honey, making them more akin to candy bars.	Homemade granola bars using nuts, seeds, and sweeteners like erythritol or monk fruit, focusing on high fiber and low net carbs.
Sweetened Condiments & Sauces	Ketchup, barbecue sauce, and salad dressings can have hidden sugars, contributing unnoticed carbs to meals.	Making homemade versions with low carb ingredients or carefully reading labels to choose brands with no added sugars.

Avoiding sugary foods and drinks is crucial on a low carb diet for several reasons. Firstly, they contribute to excessive calorie intake without providing any nutritional value, leading to weight gain and obesity. Secondly, high sugar intake is associated with spikes in blood glucose and insulin levels, which can disrupt insulin sensitivity over time and increase the risk of type 2 diabetes, heart disease, and other metabolic disorders. Lastly, reducing sugar intake can help improve overall dietary habits, leading to better health outcomes and adherence to a low carb lifestyle. By choosing low carb alternatives, individuals can enjoy delicious and satisfying options without compromising their health goals.

Grains and Starchy Foods

Food Category	Examples	Reasons to Avoid	Impact on Low Carb Diet
Grains	Wheat (including whole wheat), rice, oats, corn, barley, quinoa, rye, millet, sorghum	Grains are high in carbohydrates, which can quickly exceed the daily carb limit on a low carb diet. Even whole grains, while containing fiber, can still contribute to a significant carb intake.	Consuming grains can disrupt ketosis (if following a ketogenic diet) or hinder weight loss efforts by increasing blood sugar and insulin levels.
Bread and Baked Goods	White bread, whole wheat bread, pastries,	These foods are typically made from refined grains and added sugars, both of which are high in	They can cause spikes in blood sugar levels, leading to increased hunger and cravings, making it challenging to stick to a low carb

Food Category	Examples	Reasons to Avoid	Impact on Low Carb Diet
	cookies, muffins, cakes, pizza dough	carbohydrates. They offer little nutritional value in terms of vitamins and minerals when compared to their carb content.	diet.
Pasta and Noodles	Traditional pasta, noodles, spaghetti, macaroni (made from wheat)	Pasta and noodles are dense in carbohydrates and offer a high glycemic load, leading to rapid increases in blood sugar and insulin levels.	These foods can derail progress on a low carb diet by significantly increasing daily carb intake, making it difficult to maintain a state of ketosis or manage weight.
Cereals	Breakfast cereals, including those	Many cereals are high in added sugars and processed grains.	They can contribute to a high daily intake of carbohydrates, disrupting blood sugar

Food Category	Examples	Reasons to Avoid	Impact on Low Carb Diet
	marketed as healthy or whole grain, granola	Even cereals labeled as "whole grain" can be high in carbs and low in fiber.	control and weight management efforts on a low carb diet.
Starchy Vegetables	Potatoes, sweet potatoes, yams, peas, corn	While these vegetables contain nutrients, their high starch content translates into a high carb count, which can be counterproductive on a low carb diet.	Consuming starchy vegetables can lead to exceeding the daily carb limit, impacting blood sugar levels and hindering the body's ability to enter ketosis or burn fat efficiently.
Legumes	Beans (black, pinto, kidney), lentils,	Legumes are a good source of protein and fiber but also contain a considerable	They can be included in small portions depending on the individual's daily carb allowance; however, in

Food Category	Examples	Reasons to Avoid	Impact on Low Carb Diet
	chickpeas	amount carbohydrates.	of a strict low carb diet, their carb content may be too high to maintain ketosis or achieve desired weight loss goals.
Snack Foods	Crackers, chips, popcorn, pretzels	These snack foods are not only high in carbohydrates but also in added fats and salts, offering little nutritional benefit and a high calorie count.	They can easily lead to overconsumption, resulting in increased calorie intake and difficulty adhering to a low carb diet's carb restrictions.

Avoiding grains and starchy foods on a low carb diet is crucial due to their high carbohydrate content, which can disrupt the metabolic benefits of low carb living, such as improved blood sugar control, enhanced fat burning, and increased satiety. Opting for low carb alternatives, like vegetables, nuts, seeds, and high-quality proteins and fats, can help maintain nutritional balance while ensuring adherence to the carb restrictions of a low carb diet.

Processed Foods and Artificial Sweeteners

Processed Foods and Artificial Sweeteners	Description	Why to Avoid
Processed Meats	Includes items like bacon, sausages, hot dogs, and deli meats. Often contain additives, preservatives, and hidden carbs.	These can have added sugars and starches, increasing carb intake unknowingly. Additionally, high consumption is linked to increased risk of chronic diseases.
Low-Fat and Diet Products	Products marketed as "low fat" often replace fats with added sugars or artificial sweeteners to improve taste.	The addition of sugars and artificial ingredients can disrupt blood sugar levels and contradict the principles of a low carb diet. They may also contribute to cravings and overeating.

Processed Foods and Artificial Sweeteners	Description	Why to Avoid
Refined Grains	White bread, pasta, rice, and breakfast cereals that have been processed to remove the bran and germ, leaving mostly carbohydrate.	Refined grains are high in carbs and low in fiber. They can spike blood sugar levels, leading to energy crashes and can hamper ketosis for those on ketogenic diets.
Sugary Beverages	Sodas, fruit juices, sweetened teas, and sports drinks are high in sugars and often contain high fructose corn syrup.	These drinks are loaded with sugars, leading to quick spikes in blood sugar and insulin levels, weight gain, and an increased risk of diabetes.
"Sugar-Free" Sweets	Products like candies, jellies, and gums that are marketed as sugar-free but contain artificial sweeteners.	Although low in carbs, artificial sweeteners can maintain a craving for sweets, potentially leading to overconsumption of other carb sources. Some studies suggest they may affect gut

Processed Foods and Artificial Sweeteners	Description	Why to Avoid
		health and glucose tolerance.
Processed Snack Foods	Chips, crackers, and snack bars often contain refined grains and sugars, along with preservatives and unhealthy fats.	High in empty calories and carbs, these snacks can derail a low carb diet, contributing to weight gain and poor health outcomes. They often lack nutritional value.
Artificial Sweeteners	Non-nutritive sweeteners like aspartame, sucralose, and saccharin are used to replace sugar in diet and zero-calorie foods.	While they don't contribute carbs, their impact on appetite, gut health, and possibly glucose tolerance is still debated. They might lead to cravings and disrupt a healthy relationship with food.

Processed Foods and Artificial Sweeteners	Description	Why to Avoid
Flavored Yogurts	Often contain added sugars or artificial sweeteners to enhance taste, despite being marketed as healthy.	The added sugars increase the carb content, making them unsuitable for a low carb diet. Artificially sweetened varieties may affect cravings and satiety signals.
Frozen Dinners	Ready-to-eat meals that are convenient but can be high in added sugars, unhealthy fats, and preservatives.	Apart from hidden carbs, these meals often lack the nutritional balance of homemade food, making it difficult to manage carb intake and overall diet quality.
Vegetable Oils and Margarine	Highly processed fats that are used in many packaged foods and for cooking.	These can contain trans fats, which are harmful to heart health. While not directly related to carb content, they're associated with inflammation and chronic diseases, contradicting the health

Processed Foods and Artificial Sweeteners	Description	Why to Avoid
		benefits sought from a low carb diet.

Avoiding these foods and ingredients supports the success of a low carb diet by minimizing hidden carb sources, reducing exposure to potentially harmful additives, and fostering a healthier relationship with food. Emphasizing whole, nutrient-dense foods over processed options can lead to better health outcomes and more sustainable weight management.

Meal Planning and Recipes

Quick and Easy Low Carb Breakfast Ideas

Building a low carb meal plan is an essential step for anyone embarking on a low carb lifestyle. This strategic approach helps in managing daily carb intake, ensuring nutritional balance, and maintaining variety in your diet. A well-structured meal plan takes the guesswork out of what to eat, making it easier to stay on track with your low carb goals. Below, we outline a comprehensive guide to building a low carb meal plan, followed by a sample week-long meal plan to get you started.

Key Components of a Low Carb Meal Plan:

- **Prioritize Low Carb Vegetables:** Fill half of your plate with low carb vegetables like leafy greens (spinach, kale), cruciferous vegetables (broccoli, cauliflower), and others like zucchini, bell peppers, and asparagus. These are high in fiber and nutrients while low in carbs.

- **Incorporate Quality Protein Sources:** Each meal should include a good protein source such as chicken, beef, pork, fish, or plant-based proteins like tofu and tempeh. Protein is essential for muscle repair and satiety.

- **Choose Healthy Fats:** Include sources of healthy fats such as avocados, olive oil, nuts, seeds, and fatty fish. Fats are crucial for absorbing vitamins and providing energy.

- **Limit High Carb Foods:** Avoid or limit high carb foods such as grains, sugary snacks, fruits high in sugar, and starchy vegetables.

- **Stay Hydrated:** Drink plenty of water throughout the day, and limit sugary drinks and high-carb alcoholic beverages.

- **Plan for Snacks:** Have low carb snacks handy to prevent high carb temptations. These can include cheese, nuts, seeds, and low carb vegetables.

-

Sample 1-Week Low Carb Meal Plan:

Day	Breakfast	Lunch	Dinner	Snacks
Monday	Scrambled eggs with spinach and mushrooms	Chicken salad with mixed greens, avocado,	Grilled salmon with asparagus and side salad	Almonds; celery sticks with cream cheese

Day	Breakfast	Lunch	Dinner	Snacks
		and olive oil dressing		
Tuesday	Greek yogurt with raspberries and flaxseeds	Turkey wrap (use lettuce as wrap) with cheese and avocado	Beef stir-fry with mixed vegetables (broccoli, bell pepper, onion) over cauliflower rice	Cheese slices; cucumber slices
Wednesday	Smoothie (spinach, almond milk, peanut butter, chia seeds)	Cobb salad with hard-boiled eggs, avocado, bacon, and blue cheese	Pork chops with roasted Brussels sprouts and side salad	Hard-boiled eggs; olives
Thursday	Omelet with cheese and avocado	Tuna salad stuffed in bell peppers	Chicken Parmesan (use almond flour for breading)	Avocado slices; walnuts

Day	Breakfast	Lunch	Dinner	Snacks
			with zucchini noodles	
Friday	Cottage cheese with sliced strawberries and nuts	Beef taco salad (use low carb taco seasoning) without tortilla chips	Shrimp and broccoli alfredo (use heavy cream and Parmesan for sauce) over zucchini noodles	Pork rinds; sliced bell peppers
Saturday	Bacon and eggs	Chicken Caesar salad (no croutons)	Lamb chops with cauliflower mash and steamed green beans	Dark chocolate (>70%); macadamia nuts
Sunday	Keto pancakes (almond flour and eggs) sugar-free	Salmon with avocado salad	Low carb pizza (cauliflower crust) with cheese, tomatoes, and	Pepperoni slices; cheese crisps

Day	Breakfast	Lunch	Dinner	Snacks
	syrup		olives	

This sample meal plan is designed to provide variety and nutritional balance, incorporating a wide range of low carb foods to keep meals interesting and satisfying. It's important to adjust portion sizes and overall carb intake according to your specific goals and nutritional needs.

Building your own low carb meal plan can be a creative and enjoyable process. Use the sample plan as a template, and experiment with swapping different low carb vegetables, proteins, and fats to suit your taste preferences and nutritional requirements. Keeping a food list and recipes handy can inspire new meal ideas and help you stay committed to your low carb lifestyle.

Satisfying Low Carb Lunches

Creating satisfying low carb lunches can make adhering to a low carb lifestyle both enjoyable and sustainable. Below is a table featuring various low carb lunch ideas, complete with recipes, cooking times, and nutritional information to help guide beginners in their meal planning endeavors.

Lunch Idea	Recipe Summary	Cooking Time	Nutritional Information per Serving
Chicken Avocado Salad	Mix diced chicken breast with ripe avocado, cherry tomatoes, cucumber, and red onion. Dress with lime juice, olive oil, salt, and pepper. Serve over a bed of mixed greens.	20 mins	Calories: 350, Carbs: 8g, Protein: 25g, Fat: 26g

Lunch Idea	Recipe Summary	Cooking Time	Nutritional Information per Serving
Zucchini Noodle Stir-Fry	Spiralize zucchini into noodles. Stir-fry with sliced bell peppers, mushrooms, and shrimp in a pan with garlic, ginger, and a splash of soy sauce or tamari. Finish with a sprinkle of sesame seeds.	30 mins	Calories: 220, Carbs: 12g, Protein: 15g, Fat: 12g
Cauliflower Rice Burrito Bowl	Sauté riced cauliflower in a pan with olive oil, cumin, and chili powder. Top with grilled chicken or beef, diced tomatoes, avocado, shredded lettuce, and a dollop of sour cream. Optional: add cheese and jalapeños	25 mins	Calories: 330, Carbs: 14g, Protein: 30g, Fat: 18g

Lunch Idea	Recipe Summary	Cooking Time	Nutritional Information per Serving
	for extra flavor.		
Egg Roll in a Bowl	Cook ground pork or chicken with shredded cabbage, carrot, and onion in a pan. Season with soy sauce or tamari, garlic, and ginger. Serve hot, garnished with green onions and sesame seeds.	20 mins	Calories: 270, Carbs: 10g, Protein: 23g, Fat: 15g
Greek Salad with Grilled Chicken	Toss chopped romaine lettuce with sliced cucumber, cherry tomatoes, red onion, olives, and feta cheese. Top with	30 mins (including chicken grilling time)	Calories: 310, Carbs: 10g, Protein: 28g, Fat: 18g

Lunch Idea	Recipe Summary	Cooking Time	Nutritional Information per Serving
	grilled chicken and dress with olive oil and red wine vinegar.		
Tuna Salad Stuffed Avocados	Mix canned tuna (drained) with mayo, Dijon mustard, chopped celery, red onion, and capers. Season with salt and pepper. Halve avocados and remove the pit. Stuff the tuna salad into the avocado halves.	15 mins	Calories: 300, Carbs: 9g, Protein: 20g, Fat: 22g
Beef Lettuce Wraps	Stir-fry ground beef with minced garlic, ginger, and diced vegetables (bell peppers, mushrooms). Season with soy sauce or	25 mins	Calories: 260, Carbs: 8g, Protein: 22g, Fat: 16g

Lunch Idea	Recipe Summary	Cooking Time	Nutritional Information per Serving
	tamari and hoisin sauce. Serve in lettuce leaves, topped with sliced green onions and sesame seeds.		
Cobb Salad	Arrange a bed of mixed greens. Top with rows of hard-boiled eggs, avocado, bacon, blue cheese, grilled chicken, and cherry tomatoes. Dress with a vinaigrette of your choice.	30 mins (including egg and bacon cooking time)	Calories: 400, Carbs: 12g, Protein: 30g, Fat: 28g
Smoked Salmon and Cream Cheese Roll-Ups	Spread cream cheese on slices of smoked salmon. Add a thin strip of cucumber and avocado, then roll up tightly. Slice	15 mins	Calories: 210, Carbs: 5g, Protein: 12g, Fat: 16g

Lunch Idea	Recipe Summary	Cooking Time	Nutritional Information per Serving
	into bite-sized pieces. Optional: serve with a side of mixed greens.		
Mediterranean Veggie Bowl	Layer a bowl with spinach or mixed greens. Top with quinoa (optional for higher carb allowance), cherry tomatoes, cucumber, kalamata olives, artichoke hearts, feta cheese, and hummus. Drizzle with olive oil and lemon juice. Serve cold or at room temperature.	20 mins (if including quinoa, add cooking time accordingly)	Calories: 320, Carbs: 18g (adjust if adding quinoa), Protein: 10g, Fat: 24g

Note: The nutritional information provided is approximate and can vary based on specific ingredients and portion sizes used.

These lunch ideas offer a balance of protein, healthy fats, and low carb vegetables, designed to fit seamlessly into a low carb dietary pattern.

Delicious Low Carb Dinners

Below is a table that includes a range of dinner ideas, each accompanied by a simple recipe, cooking time, and basic nutritional information to help beginners plan their meals efficiently. These recipes focus on incorporating low carb vegetables, lean proteins, and healthy fats to ensure each meal is both satisfying and aligned with low carb dietary goals.

Dinner Idea	Recipe	Cooking Time	Nutritional Information (per serving)
Zucchini Lasagna	**Ingredients:** 2 large zucchinis (sliced thin), 1 lb ground beef, 1 cup marinara sauce (low sugar), 1 cup ricotta cheese, 1 egg, 1 cup shredded mozzarella, salt, and pepper. **Instructions:** Brown beef, layer zucchini, meat, mixed ricotta & egg, sauce, and mozzarella. Repeat. Bake at 375°F for 45 minutes.	60 minutes	Calories: 320, Carbs: 12g, Protein: 25g, Fat: 20g
Cauliflower	**Ingredients:** 1 head cauliflower	30	Calories:

Dinner Idea	Recipe	Cooking Time	Nutritional Information (per serving)
Crust Pizza	(riced and drained), 1 egg, ½ cup mozzarella, 2 tsp Italian seasoning, toppings of choice. **Instructions:** Mix cauliflower, egg, cheese, and seasoning. Form into a crust on a baking sheet. Bake at 425°F for 20 minutes. Add toppings, bake until cheese melts.	minutes	150, Carbs: 10g, Protein: 10g, Fat: 8g
Grilled Salmon with Asparagus	**Ingredients:** 4 salmon fillets, 1 lb asparagus, 2 tbsp olive oil, lemon wedges, salt, and pepper. **Instructions:** Season salmon and asparagus. Grill over medium-high heat, salmon for 4 minutes per side and asparagus for 6-8 minutes, until tender. Serve with lemon.	20 minutes	Calories: 350, Carbs: 6g, Protein: 34g, Fat: 22g
Chicken Stir-Fry with Broccoli	**Ingredients:** 1 lb chicken breast (sliced), 2 cups broccoli florets, 1 bell pepper (sliced), 2 tbsp soy sauce (low sodium), 1 tbsp olive	25 minutes	Calories: 280, Carbs: 8g, Protein: 27g, Fat: 16g

Dinner Idea	Recipe	Cooking Time	Nutritional Information (per serving)
	oil, garlic, and ginger. **Instructions:** Stir-fry chicken in oil until browned. Add vegetables, soy sauce, garlic, and ginger. Cook until vegetables are tender.		
Beef and Vegetable Skillet	**Ingredients:** 1 lb lean ground beef, 1 cup diced bell peppers, 1 cup spinach, 1 cup mushrooms, 2 tbsp taco seasoning, 1 avocado (diced), 1 tbsp olive oil. **Instructions:** Brown beef in oil, add vegetables and seasoning. Cook until veggies are soft. Top with avocado.	20 minutes	Calories: 300, Carbs: 12g, Protein: 23g, Fat: 18g
Shrimp and Zoodle Alfredo	**Ingredients:** 1 lb shrimp (peeled), 4 zucchinis (spiraled), 1 cup Alfredo sauce (low carb), 1 tbsp olive oil, parmesan cheese. **Instructions:** Sauté shrimp in oil until pink. Add zoodles, cook until	20 minutes	Calories: 330, Carbs: 8g, Protein: 28g, Fat: 22g

Dinner Idea	Recipe	Cooking Time	Nutritional Information (per serving)
	soft. Stir in Alfredo sauce, heat through. Top with parmesan.		
Stuffed Bell Peppers	**Ingredients:** 4 bell peppers (halved and seeded), 1 lb ground turkey, 1 cup cauliflower rice, 1 cup diced tomatoes (drained), 1 tsp cumin, 1 tsp chili powder, 1 cup shredded cheese. **Instructions:** Mix turkey, cauliflower rice, tomatoes, spices. Stuff peppers, top with cheese. Bake at 375°F for 30 min.	45 minutes	Calories: 240, Carbs: 12g, Protein: 21g, Fat: 12g

These dinner ideas are designed to fit seamlessly into a low carb diet, providing a mix of flavors and nutrients that support a healthy lifestyle without compromising on taste. By incorporating a variety of vegetables, lean proteins, and healthy fats, these recipes ensure that you can enjoy delicious dinners that help you stay on track with your low carb goals. Each recipe is straightforward, making it easy to expand their culinary skills and enjoy a diverse diet.

Low Carb Snacks and Desserts

Below is a table featuring a selection of low carb snack and dessert ideas, complete with recipes, cooking times, and nutritional information. These options are designed to satisfy cravings without compromising your low carb lifestyle.

Snack/Dessert	Recipe Highlights	Cooking Time	Nutritional Information (per serving)
Almond Flour Chocolate Chip Cookies	Mix 2 cups almond flour, 1/2 cup erythritol, 1 tsp baking powder, 1/4 cup melted butter, 2 tsp vanilla extract, and 1/2 cup sugar-free chocolate chips. Drop spoonfuls onto a baking sheet and bake.	12-15 min at 350°F	Calories: 160, Carbs: 5g (Net Carbs: 2g), Protein: 5g, Fat: 14g

Snack/Dessert	Recipe Highlights	Cooking Time	Nutritional Information (per serving)
Cheese Crisps	Place small piles of shredded cheese on a baking sheet lined with parchment paper. Season with spices if desired. Bake until crispy.	6-8 min at 400°F	Calories: 100, Carbs: 1g, Protein: 7g, Fat: 8g
Avocado Chocolate Mousse	Blend 1 ripe avocado, 1/4 cup cocoa powder, 1/4 cup almond milk, 1/4 cup erythritol, and 1 tsp vanilla extract until smooth. Chill before serving.	No cook, chill for 1 hour	Calories: 120, Carbs: 8g (Net Carbs: 3g), Protein: 2g, Fat: 10g
Cauliflower Buffalo Bites	Toss cauliflower florets with olive oil and bake. Once tender, coat with a mixture of hot sauce and melted butter and bake again until crispy.	25-30 min at 425°F	Calories: 150, Carbs: 10g (Net Carbs: 6g), Protein: 3g, Fat: 11g

Snack/Dessert	Recipe Highlights	Cooking Time	Nutritional Information (per serving)
Zucchini Chips	Slice zucchini thinly, season with salt, and lay on a baking sheet. Bake until crispy. Optional: sprinkle with Parmesan in the last few minutes of baking.	1-2 hours at 225°F	Calories: 50, Carbs: 4g (Net Carbs: 3g), Protein: 2g, Fat: 4g
Peanut Butter Fat Bombs	Mix 1 cup natural peanut butter (no sugar added), 1/4 cup coconut oil, and 1/4 cup erythritol. Pour into molds and freeze.	No cook, freeze for 2 hours	Calories: 200, Carbs: 5g (Net Carbs: 3g), Protein: 6g, Fat: 18g
Berry and Cream Cheese Bites	Mix 1/4 cup cream cheese with 1 tbsp erythritol. Spoon a small amount onto a raspberry or strawberry half and top with a nut or chocolate piece.	No cook	Calories: 30, Carbs: 2g (Net Carbs: 1g), Protein: 1g, Fat: 2g

Snack/Dessert	Recipe Highlights	Cooking Time	Nutritional Information (per serving)
Cucumber and Salmon Bites	Slice cucumber into rounds. Top each with a small slice of smoked salmon, a dollop of cream cheese, and a sprinkle of dill.	No cook	Calories: 20, Carbs: 1g, Protein: 3g, Fat: 1g

These snack and dessert ideas showcase how a low carb diet can still include a wide variety of tasty options. By focusing on low carb ingredients and healthy fats, you can enjoy indulgent flavors without the guilt. Remember, portion control is key, even with low carb treats, to ensure you stay within your daily macronutrient goals. Enjoy exploring these recipes as part of your meal planning and discover how satisfying low carb eating can be!

Eating Out and Social Events

Navigating Restaurants on a Low Carb Diet

Eating out while following a low carb diet can present a challenge, but with a bit of planning and savvy decision-making, it's entirely possible to enjoy social events and restaurant meals without straying from your dietary goals. The key lies in understanding menu options, making informed choices, and not being afraid to ask for modifications to suit your low carb lifestyle.

Before heading to a restaurant, doing some research can significantly improve your dining experience. Many establishments offer their menus online, providing an opportunity to review options and decide what to eat ahead of time. Look for dishes that are rich in proteins and vegetables, and low in carbohydrates. Salads, grilled meats, and seafood are often good choices, but watch out for dressings, sauces, and marinades that can contain hidden sugars and carbs.

When in doubt, don't hesitate to ask your server about the ingredients in a dish. Chefs typically aim to accommodate dietary restrictions, and a simple request can often result in a meal that fits within your low carb parameters. For instance, asking for a burger without the bun or swapping out a side of fries for a salad are easy modifications that most restaurants are willing to make.

Beverages can also be a hidden source of carbs. Opt for water, unsweetened tea, or coffee, and avoid sugary drinks and alcohol, which can add a significant amount of carbohydrates to your meal. If you choose to drink alcohol, select options with lower carb contents like dry wine or spirits mixed with zero-carb mixers.

Appetizers and shared plates offer an opportunity to control your intake by choosing low carb options like meat and cheese platters, vegetables with dip, or seafood starters. Avoid bread baskets, chips, and other carb-heavy starters that are often placed on the table before the meal.

Understanding portion sizes can also help you manage your carb intake. Restaurant portions are typically larger than standard serving sizes, so consider sharing a dish or asking for half of your meal to be boxed up before you begin eating. This strategy can help you avoid overeating and inadvertently consuming too many carbs.

Desserts can be the most challenging part of dining out on a low carb diet. If you're tempted by sweet endings, look for cheese selections, berries with cream (ask for it unsweetened), or simply opt for a cup of coffee to conclude your meal. Many people find that their craving for sweets diminishes after adopting a low carb lifestyle, so skipping dessert may become easier over time.

Finally, embracing flexibility is crucial when eating out on a low carb diet. While it's important to stick to your dietary goals, occasional deviations are part of a balanced lifestyle. If you find that your options are limited, choose the best available dish and enjoy the social experience without guilt. One meal won't derail your progress, and you can always return to stricter low carb eating with your next meal.

Navigating restaurants on a low carb diet becomes easier with practice. By making informed choices, asking for modifications, and focusing on the enjoyment of socializing over the stress of dietary restrictions, you can maintain your low carb lifestyle without missing out on the pleasures of dining out.

Low Carb Alcohol and Beverages

Navigating social events and dining out can pose a challenge for those following a low carb diet, especially when it comes to choosing the right beverages. Alcohol and many popular drinks often contain hidden sugars and carbs, which can easily derail dietary goals. However, with the right knowledge, you can enjoy social gatherings without compromising your low carb lifestyle.

When it comes to alcohol, the key is to choose drinks with lower carb content. Spirits such as vodka, rum, gin, tequila, and whiskey are virtually carb-free by themselves. However, mixing these with sodas or juice can add significant amounts of sugar and carbs. Opting for mixers like club soda, diet tonic, or simply adding a slice of lime or lemon can keep your drink low in carbs. Dry wines, both red and white, offer another viable option as they contain minimal sugars. It's advisable to avoid sweet wines, dessert wines, and most beer, as these are typically high in carbs.

Light beers and certain craft beers that are marketed as low carb could be acceptable in moderation, but it's important to check their carb content as it can vary. Seltzers, particularly those without added sugar, are also a good low carb choice, offering a variety of flavors without the carb load of traditional flavored beverages.

Beyond alcohol, beverages such as coffee and tea are naturally low in carbs and can be enjoyed freely on a low carb diet. However, additions like sugar, milk, and flavored syrups can increase the carb count significantly. Switching to heavy cream or unsweetened almond or coconut milk can make your coffee or tea more diet-friendly. For those who prefer their drinks sweetened, consider using stevia or erythritol, which are natural sweeteners that do not affect blood sugar levels.

Water should be the cornerstone of hydration for everyone, especially those on a low carb diet. Infusing water with cucumber, berries, or citrus can add flavor without the carbs found in fruit juices and soda. Carbonated mineral water is another excellent option, providing the satisfaction of a fizzy drink without the sugar and carbs of soft drinks.

Diet sodas and other sugar-free beverages can fit into a low carb lifestyle, but it's essential to consume them in moderation. While they don't contain sugar or carbs, the artificial sweeteners in these drinks can sometimes trigger cravings for sweet foods and disrupt metabolic health in some individuals.

In social settings, being mindful of your beverage choices can help you stay on track with your low carb diet. Planning ahead and knowing which drinks to choose can make eating out and attending events less stressful and more enjoyable. Remember, the focus should be on enjoying the company and the experience rather than worrying about dietary restrictions. With a bit of preparation and knowledge, you can navigate any social situation without compromising your health goals.

Handling Social Gatherings and Holidays

Handling social gatherings and holidays can be one of the more challenging aspects of maintaining a low carb diet, but with the right strategies, it's entirely possible to enjoy these events without compromising your dietary goals. Social settings often revolve around food, and these foods are not always compatible with a low carb lifestyle. However, preparation, communication, and smart choices can help you navigate these situations successfully.

Firstly, being prepared is crucial. If you're aware of a social gathering or holiday event in advance, consider eating a small, low carb meal or snack before attending. This can help curb hunger, making it easier to resist high carb temptations. Another effective strategy is to bring a low carb dish to share. This ensures there will be at least one item you can enjoy without worry, and it also introduces others to the delicious possibilities of low carb eating.

When dining out, don't hesitate to ask for modifications to your meal. Most restaurants are willing to accommodate dietary requests, such as substituting high carb sides like fries or mashed potatoes with vegetables or a salad. Additionally, focusing on dishes that naturally align with a low carb diet, such as grilled meats and seafood, can make dining out less stressful.

Beverages can also be a source of hidden carbs. Opt for water, unsweetened tea, or coffee, and be cautious with alcohol, as many cocktails contain high amounts of sugar. If you choose to drink, select lower carb options like dry wine or spirits with zero carb mixers like club soda.

During holidays, traditional foods often hold significant emotional and cultural importance, making it particularly challenging to stick to dietary restrictions. In these instances, it's helpful to focus on portion control. Allowing yourself a small taste of higher carb foods can satisfy cravings without derailing your diet. Remember, moderation is key.

Another strategy is to prioritize protein and vegetables on your plate. This can help you feel full and satisfied, reducing the temptation to overindulge in high carb dishes. Also, consider starting new traditions with low carb alternatives that are just as satisfying as their high carb counterparts. Many traditional recipes can be modified to fit a low carb profile without sacrificing flavor.

It's also important to communicate with your hosts or fellow guests about your dietary needs. People are often accommodating once they understand your health goals. However, it's equally important to be gracious and flexible. If you end up consuming more carbs than planned, don't be too hard on yourself. One meal won't ruin your progress, and it's crucial to enjoy these moments of connection and celebration.

Finally, staying mindful of your eating during social events can help you make better food choices. Engaging in conversations and savoring each bite can prevent mindless eating and help you enjoy the experience more fully.

By employing these strategies, social gatherings and holidays can still be enjoyable and fulfilling aspects of your life, even on a low carb diet. Preparation, smart choices, and a balanced approach to eating can ensure that you stay on track with your dietary goals while still making the most of these special occasions.

Monitoring Your Progress

Tracking Your Carb Intake

Tracking your carb intake is an essential aspect of following a low carb diet, especially . It not only helps you stay within your daily carb limit but also enables you to understand how different foods affect your body and weight loss journey. With a myriad of tools and strategies at your disposal, keeping an eye on your carbs can be simplified, making it easier to achieve your health and wellness goals.

Starting with the basics, keeping a food diary is a straightforward method to monitor your carb intake. This can be as simple as jotting down what you eat in a notebook or using a digital app. The key is to be consistent and detailed, recording everything you consume, including snacks and beverages, as these can add up. When you write down your meals, make sure to note the portion sizes and the estimated carb content. This practice helps you become more aware of your eating habits and the carb values of different foods, aiding in making better dietary choices.

Digital apps provide a more advanced way to track your carb intake. Many of these apps come with extensive databases of foods, including generic items, branded products, and restaurant dishes, making it easier to log what you eat accurately. They often calculate your daily totals for carbs, fiber, protein, and fat, offering insights into your overall nutritional balance. Some apps also allow you to set goals, track your progress over time, and provide reports that you can share with a nutritionist or doctor for further advice.

Another effective strategy is to use a food scale, at least initially, until you get a good sense of portion sizes. Weighing your food and referring to the nutritional information can provide a more accurate estimate of your carb intake, which is particularly useful for foods that are easy to overeat, such as nuts and cheeses.

For those who enjoy cooking or meal prep, calculating the total carbs in homemade meals can be done by adding up the carb content of the individual ingredients. Divide this total by the number of servings the recipe yields to find out the carbs per serving. This might require a bit of math, but it becomes more intuitive over time.

As you track your carb intake, it's important to focus on net carbs, which are calculated by subtracting the grams of fiber from the total grams of carbs. Since fiber doesn't raise blood sugar levels in the same way other carbohydrates do, focusing on net carbs can provide a more accurate measure of how a food impacts your diet.

Paying attention to how you feel and how your body responds to different levels of carb intake is also vital. Some people may need to adjust their carb threshold to continue losing weight or to address specific health concerns. Regularly reviewing your food diary or app entries can help you identify patterns, triggers for cravings, or foods that don't satisfy you, allowing for adjustments to your diet plan.

Lastly, consistency is key when tracking your carb intake. It might seem tedious at first, but it becomes a valuable habit that can significantly contribute to your success on a low carb diet. Whether you choose a pen and paper, a digital app, or a combination of methods, the goal is to find a system that works for you and stick with it. This diligent approach to monitoring your carb intake can lead to a deeper understanding of your dietary needs and help you make lasting changes to your eating habits.

Understanding Weight Fluctuations

Understanding weight fluctuations is crucial for anyone on a low carb diet, as it can significantly impact how you perceive your progress and maintain motivation. Many beginners expect a steady decrease in weight when they embark on a low carb journey, but the reality is that weight can fluctuate daily due to a variety of factors. Recognizing these factors and learning not to be discouraged by them is key to a successful and sustainable low carb lifestyle.

First and foremost, water retention plays a major role in weight fluctuations. Carbohydrates are stored in the body along with water; when you reduce your carb intake, you also reduce water retention, leading to rapid weight loss in the initial stages of a low carb diet. However, this process can reverse slightly when you reintroduce or increase carbs, leading to temporary weight gain, not necessarily fat. This is why monitoring carb intake closely and understanding its direct impact on water retention is important.

Hydration levels also affect weight fluctuations. Being well-hydrated is crucial for your body to function optimally, especially on a low carb diet. However, your hydration status can cause your weight to vary from day to day. For example, dehydration can lead to a temporary drop in weight, while drinking plenty of water can cause a temporary increase. This doesn't reflect changes in body fat but rather the amount of water your body is holding onto at any given time.

Another factor is the natural variance in food intake and digestion. The weight of the food and liquid you consume throughout the day doesn't instantly disappear; it's processed, absorbed, or excreted by your body over time. Consequently, eating a large meal or more salt than usual can lead to temporary weight gains due to increased food volume and water retention from higher sodium intake.

Exercise and physical activity can also lead to misleading weight fluctuations. After intense exercise, especially strength training, your muscles may retain water to aid in recovery. While this is a positive sign of your body responding to the exercise, it can also temporarily reflect as weight gain on the scale.

Hormonal changes, particularly in women, can cause significant weight fluctuations. Hormones regulate water retention, and fluctuations during menstrual cycles can lead to temporary weight gain. Additionally, stress hormones like cortisol can impact weight by promoting water retention and influencing eating habits.

Understanding these factors is essential for anyone on a low carb diet. It's important to focus on long-term trends rather than daily numbers. Using a combination of metrics to monitor progress, such as measurements, how clothes fit, energy levels, and overall health improvements, can provide a more comprehensive view of your success.

Moreover, recognizing that weight fluctuations are normal and part of the process helps in adjusting the diet as needed and avoiding unnecessary frustration. Instead of getting discouraged by temporary changes, it's beneficial to stay consistent with the low carb lifestyle, trust the process, and focus on making healthy choices that support your overall goals. This approach not only leads to sustainable weight loss but also contributes to improved health and well-being in the long run.

Adjusting Your Diet for Ongoing Success

Adjusting your diet for ongoing success is a dynamic process that requires attention to your body's responses, the ability to recognize when changes are needed, and the knowledge to implement those changes effectively. In the context of a low carb diet, this means closely monitoring your progress, understanding the impact of different foods on your body, and being willing to make necessary adjustments to ensure continued success and health improvement.

One of the first steps in adjusting your diet for ongoing success is to keep a detailed food diary. Recording what you eat, when you eat, and how you feel afterwards can provide invaluable insights into how different foods affect your energy levels, mood, hunger, and overall well-being. This practice can help you identify patterns or specific foods that may not be conducive to your goals, allowing you to make more informed decisions about your diet.

Understanding the nuances of your body's responses to different types of foods is crucial. For instance, some people may find that they can tolerate higher amounts of natural carbohydrates from vegetables or dairy without impacting their weight loss or health goals. Others might discover that even small amounts of certain carbs can stall their progress. Listening to your body and adjusting your carb intake accordingly is key to finding the balance that works best for you.

Experimentation plays a vital role in adjusting your diet for ongoing success. This could mean experimenting with the timing of your meals, such as incorporating intermittent fasting, or adjusting the macronutrient ratios of your meals to see what combination makes you feel best. Some individuals thrive on a higher fat intake, while others may need more protein to feel satiated and maintain muscle mass.

As you progress on your low carb journey, it's important to revisit and possibly redefine your goals. Weight loss might have been your initial motivation, but over time, your focus might shift towards maintaining your weight, improving athletic performance, or enhancing overall health markers like blood sugar levels and cholesterol levels. These evolving goals may necessitate adjustments in your diet. For example, increasing your carb intake slightly can provide additional energy for intense workouts, while still keeping you within the low carb range.

Monitoring your progress extends beyond the scale. Using other metrics such as body measurements, energy levels, sleep quality, and blood markers can provide a more comprehensive picture of your health and the effectiveness of your diet. These indicators can help guide your dietary adjustments, ensuring that you're not only losing weight but also improving your overall health.

Education is an ongoing part of adjusting your diet for success. Keeping informed about the latest research and recommendations for low carb eating can introduce you to new foods, supplements, and strategies that might be beneficial for your specific situation. Engaging with the low carb community, whether online or in person, can also provide support, inspiration, and practical tips for navigating challenges and making effective adjustments to your diet.

In summary, adjusting your diet for ongoing success on a low carb plan involves a combination of self-monitoring, listening to your body, being open to experimentation, and staying informed. By paying close attention to how your body responds to different foods and making adjustments based on what you learn, you can maintain progress towards your goals, overcome plateaus, and ensure that your diet continues to meet your evolving needs for health and well-being.

Overcoming Challenges

Managing Cravings

Managing cravings is a pivotal aspect of successfully navigating a low carb diet, especially who might find the transition challenging. Cravings for high-carb foods like sweets, bread, pasta, and rice can become significant hurdles. However, understanding the roots of these cravings and employing strategies to handle them can make the journey smoother and more sustainable.

Firstly, it's essential to distinguish between physical hunger and emotional cravings. Physical hunger gradually builds and can be satisfied with various foods, whereas cravings are often sudden and specific. Recognizing this difference is key to managing cravings effectively.

One effective strategy is ensuring you're consuming enough whole, nutrient-dense foods. A common mistake is not eating enough fats and proteins, which are crucial on a low carb diet. These macronutrients are satiating and can significantly reduce cravings by stabilizing blood sugar levels and promoting a feeling of fullness.

Another tactic involves hydration. Sometimes, the body can misinterpret dehydration as hunger. Drinking water, especially before meals, can help mitigate this and reduce unnecessary snacking. Incorporating beverages like herbal tea or flavored water can also provide a satisfying alternative to high-carb drinks.

Cravings often have a psychological component, where certain foods are associated with comfort or reward. Finding low carb alternatives that satisfy these emotional connections can be incredibly effective. For instance, using cauliflower as a substitute for mashed potatoes or making zucchini noodles instead of pasta allows for the enjoyment of familiar dishes without the high carb content.

Regular physical activity is another tool for managing cravings. Exercise not only helps in maintaining a healthy weight but also in reducing stress and improving mood, which can lessen the frequency and intensity of cravings. Even light activities like walking or yoga can have a positive impact.

Sleep plays a critical role in managing cravings. Lack of sleep can increase hunger hormone levels and decrease satiety hormone levels, leading to increased appetite and cravings. Ensuring adequate, quality sleep can help keep these hormones in balance and reduce cravings.

Mindful eating practices can also aid in managing cravings. Eating slowly and without distractions allows the body to recognize fullness cues, reducing the likelihood of overeating or giving in to cravings. It also enhances the enjoyment of food, making satisfying meals with fewer carbs more fulfilling.

For moments when cravings do arise, having a plan in place can make all the difference. Keeping healthy, low carb snacks on hand can prevent reaching for high-carb options. Snacks high in fiber, protein, or healthy fats, like nuts, seeds, or cheese, can be particularly effective.

Finally, allowing for occasional, controlled indulgence can help manage cravings without derailing dietary goals. Incorporating a small serving of a craved item into your diet plan occasionally can prevent feelings of deprivation that might lead to bingeing.

Managing cravings on a low carb diet involves a combination of strategies focusing on diet composition, lifestyle adjustments, psychological understanding, and mindful indulgence. By employing these tactics, individuals can overcome one of the most common challenges in low carb eating, paving the way for a healthier, more satisfying dietary lifestyle.

Plateaus: Why They Happen and What to Do

Plateaus are a common challenge encountered by individuals following a low carb diet. After experiencing initial success in weight loss and improvements in health, it's not uncommon to reach a point where progress stalls, and the scale refuses to budge. Understanding why plateaus happen and how to overcome them is crucial for maintaining motivation and achieving long-term success on a low carb journey.

One reason for plateaus is metabolic adaptation. When you reduce your carb intake, your body adjusts its metabolism to conserve energy, making weight loss more challenging over time. This is a natural response to prolonged calorie restriction and can lead to a plateau in weight loss. Additionally, as you lose weight, your body requires fewer calories to maintain its current weight, further slowing down your metabolism.

Another factor contributing to plateaus is the body's tendency to reach a state of equilibrium, also known as homeostasis. As you consistently follow a low carb diet, your body may adapt to the new dietary pattern, resulting in a temporary halt in weight loss. This can be frustrating, especially if you've been diligently adhering to your meal plan and exercise routine.

Moreover, plateaus can occur due to factors beyond diet and exercise, such as stress, lack of sleep, hormonal fluctuations, and medication side effects. These external influences can impact your body's ability to burn fat efficiently, making it more challenging to break through a weight loss plateau.

So, what can you do to overcome plateaus and continue making progress on your low carb journey? Firstly, it's essential to reassess your dietary habits and make adjustments as needed. This may involve tracking your food intake more diligently, reducing portion sizes, or incorporating intermittent fasting to kickstart fat burning.

Additionally, varying your exercise routine can help revitalize your metabolism and break through plateaus. Incorporating strength training exercises can build lean muscle mass, which in turn boosts your metabolism and enhances fat burning. High-intensity interval training (HIIT) is another effective approach for overcoming plateaus, as it elevates your heart rate and promotes calorie burning long after the workout is complete.

Furthermore, paying attention to non-scale victories can provide motivation during plateaus. Focus on improvements in energy levels, sleep quality, mood, and overall well-being, rather than solely relying on the number on the scale. Celebrate small achievements and milestones along the way to stay motivated and committed to your low carb lifestyle.

Lastly, be patient and persistent. Plateaus are a normal part of the weight loss journey, and breaking through them requires time, dedication, and consistency. Stay focused on your goals, trust the process, and remember that setbacks are temporary. With perseverance and the right strategies in place, you can overcome plateaus and continue progressing towards your health and wellness goals on your low carb journey.

Balancing Exercise with a Low Carb Diet

When adopting a low carb diet, many individuals may wonder about the role of exercise in conjunction with their dietary changes. Balancing exercise with a low carb diet can be a key component of achieving overall health and weight management goals, but it requires careful consideration and understanding of how these two elements interact.

First and foremost, it's essential to recognize that exercise and nutrition are interconnected aspects of a healthy lifestyle. While diet plays a significant role in weight loss and metabolic health, regular physical activity offers numerous benefits beyond just burning calories. Exercise helps build and maintain lean muscle mass, improves cardiovascular health, enhances mood, and boosts overall energy levels.

When combining exercise with a low carb diet, it's important to consider timing and intensity. Depending on individual preferences and goals, different types of exercise may be more suitable. For instance, low to moderate-intensity activities such as walking, cycling, or yoga can complement a low carb diet by promoting overall well-being and aiding in weight management without significantly increasing carbohydrate demands.

High-intensity exercises, such as interval training or weightlifting, can also be compatible with a low carb diet, but they may require adjustments in timing and fueling strategies. Since high-intensity workouts rely heavily on glycogen stores for energy, individuals following a low carb diet may need to ensure adequate glycogen replenishment before engaging in such activities. This can be achieved by strategically timing carbohydrate intake around workouts or consuming small amounts of easily digestible carbs pre-exercise to provide immediate energy.

Moreover, it's essential to listen to your body and adjust your exercise routine accordingly when following a low carb diet. Some individuals may experience a temporary decrease in exercise performance during the initial stages of carbohydrate restriction as the body adapts to using fat for fuel instead of carbohydrates. This phenomenon, often referred to as the "low carb flu," typically resolves within a few days to weeks as the body becomes more efficient at utilizing fat stores for energy.

To mitigate any potential negative effects on exercise performance while transitioning to a low carb diet, it's crucial to prioritize hydration, electrolyte balance, and sufficient rest. Staying hydrated and replenishing electrolytes, especially sodium, potassium, and magnesium, can help alleviate symptoms of fatigue, muscle cramps, and dizziness commonly associated with the initial stages of carbohydrate restriction.

Furthermore, incorporating adequate protein and healthy fats into your diet can support muscle repair and recovery, ensuring that your body has the nutrients it needs to sustain physical activity while following a low carb eating plan. Consuming protein-rich foods such as lean meats, poultry, fish, eggs, and plant-based sources like tofu, tempeh, and legumes can help maintain muscle mass and promote exercise performance.

Balancing exercise with a low carb diet requires careful attention to individual needs, preferences, and goals. By choosing the right types of exercise, timing workouts strategically, and prioritizing proper nutrition and hydration, individuals can maximize the benefits of both exercise and dietary changes for overall health and well-being.

Advanced Low Carb Strategies

Intermittent Fasting and Low Carb Synergy

Intermittent fasting (IF) and a low carb diet are two dietary strategies that have gained popularity for their potential health benefits, including weight loss, improved metabolic health, and increased longevity. When combined, these two approaches can synergize to enhance their individual effects, leading to greater results for those seeking to optimize their health and wellness.

Intermittent fasting involves cycling between periods of eating and fasting. The most common IF protocols include the 16/8 method, where individuals fast for 16 hours and consume all their meals within an 8-hour window, and the 5:2 method, where individuals eat normally for five days of the week and restrict calorie intake on the remaining two days.

When paired with a low carb diet, intermittent fasting can amplify the metabolic benefits associated with both approaches. By reducing carbohydrate intake, particularly refined carbohydrates and sugars, the body is encouraged to burn fat for fuel instead of relying on glucose derived from carbohydrates. This metabolic shift promotes ketosis, a state where the body produces ketones from fat breakdown, which can lead to increased fat burning and weight loss.

During fasting periods, insulin levels decrease, allowing the body to access stored fat for energy more efficiently. Since low carb diets also help stabilize blood sugar levels and reduce insulin spikes, the combination of IF and low carb eating can further enhance insulin sensitivity, which is beneficial for overall metabolic health and may reduce the risk of type 2 diabetes.

Moreover, intermittent fasting can complement the appetite-suppressing effects of a low carb diet, making it easier to adhere to reduced calorie intake without feeling deprived. By extending the fasting window, individuals may naturally consume fewer calories overall, leading to greater weight loss and fat loss over time.

Intermittent fasting and a low carb diet also have synergistic effects on other aspects of health, such as inflammation and cellular repair processes. Studies have shown that both approaches can reduce markers of inflammation in the body, which are linked to various chronic diseases, including heart disease and cancer. Additionally, intermittent fasting has been shown to promote autophagy, a cellular cleansing process that removes damaged cells and promotes cellular rejuvenation.

While intermittent fasting and a low carb diet can offer significant benefits when combined, it's essential to approach this strategy with caution, especially or individuals with specific health conditions. It's crucial to listen to your body's signals and adjust your fasting and eating windows accordingly to ensure you're meeting your nutritional needs and maintaining overall well-being.

In conclusion, intermittent fasting and a low carb diet can synergize to enhance weight loss, metabolic health, and overall well-being. By reducing carbohydrate intake and incorporating periods of fasting, individuals may experience greater fat burning, improved insulin sensitivity, and reduced inflammation. However, it's essential to approach this strategy mindfully and consult with a healthcare professional if you have any concerns or underlying health conditions.

Ketogenic Diet: Taking Low Carb to the Next Level

The ketogenic diet, often referred to as keto, is a low carb, high fat diet that takes the principles of low carb eating to the next level. It's designed to transition the body into a state of ketosis, where it primarily burns fat for fuel instead of carbohydrates. This metabolic shift can have profound effects on weight loss, energy levels, and overall health, making it an attractive option for those seeking advanced low carb strategies.

The key principle of the ketogenic diet is drastically reducing carbohydrate intake while increasing fat consumption. By restricting carbs to around 20-50 grams per day, the body is deprived of its primary source of energy, prompting it to enter ketosis. In this state, the liver converts fat into ketones, which serve as an alternative fuel source for the body and brain.

To achieve and maintain ketosis, it's essential to choose foods that are not only low in carbs but also high in healthy fats. This includes foods like avocados, nuts, seeds, olive oil, fatty fish, and coconut oil. These fats provide sustained energy and help keep you feeling full and satisfied, making it easier to stick to the ketogenic diet long-term.

Protein intake is also moderated on the ketogenic diet to prevent excess gluconeogenesis, a process where the body converts protein into glucose, potentially disrupting ketosis. While protein is still an essential component of the diet for muscle repair and other bodily functions, it's important to choose moderate portions of high-quality protein sources such as meat, poultry, fish, and eggs.

While the ketogenic diet primarily focuses on reducing carbs and increasing fats, it's important to prioritize nutrient-dense foods to ensure overall health and wellbeing. This means incorporating plenty of non-starchy vegetables, leafy greens, and other low carb, high fiber foods to provide essential vitamins, minerals, and antioxidants.

One of the most significant benefits of the ketogenic diet is its potential for weight loss and fat loss. By shifting the body's metabolism away from relying on carbohydrates for energy, it becomes more efficient at burning stored fat for fuel. This can lead to rapid weight loss, especially in the initial stages of the diet.

In addition to weight loss, the ketogenic diet has been shown to have numerous other health benefits. Research suggests it may improve blood sugar control, reduce inflammation, lower triglyceride levels, and even improve cognitive function in some individuals.

However, it's essential to approach the ketogenic diet with caution, especially if you have underlying health conditions or are taking medications. It's always advisable to consult with a healthcare professional before making significant dietary changes, especially those as drastic as the ketogenic diet.

In conclusion, the ketogenic diet offers a powerful approach to low carb eating, taking it to the next level by promoting ketosis and fat adaptation. By drastically reducing carbohydrate intake and increasing healthy fat consumption, individuals can experience significant weight loss, improved energy levels, and numerous other health benefits. However, it's essential to approach the ketogenic diet with knowledge, caution, and guidance to ensure safety and long-term success.

Carb Cycling for Enhanced Fat Loss

Carb cycling is an advanced dietary strategy that involves alternating between high and low carbohydrate intake over specific periods. This approach is often used by athletes, bodybuilders, and fitness enthusiasts to optimize fat loss while preserving muscle mass and performance. While it may not be suitable for everyone, carb cycling can be a powerful tool for those looking to enhance their fat loss efforts within the framework of a low carb diet.

The concept behind carb cycling revolves around manipulating carbohydrate intake to exploit its impact on hormones and metabolism. By cycling between periods of low carb intake (often referred to as "low carb days") and higher carb intake ("refeed days" or "high carb days"), individuals aim to maximize fat burning while mitigating the potential negative effects of prolonged carbohydrate restriction.

During low carb days, carbohydrate intake is significantly reduced, typically to less than 50 grams per day or even lower. This forces the body to rely primarily on fat stores for energy, promoting fat loss and ketosis, a metabolic state where the body burns fat for fuel instead of carbohydrates. Low carb days are often paired with higher protein and moderate to higher fat intake to support muscle maintenance and satiety.

Refeed or high carb days, on the other hand, involve strategically increasing carbohydrate intake, usually to levels that match or slightly exceed daily energy expenditure. This temporary increase in carbs replenishes glycogen stores, boosts energy levels, and stimulates the release of hormones like leptin, which can help prevent metabolic slowdown and maintain thyroid function. Refeed days are typically scheduled around intense workouts or as a periodic break from the low carb regimen.

The key to successful carb cycling lies in careful planning and timing. It's essential to tailor the cycling schedule to individual goals, activity levels, and metabolic responses. Some may benefit from a more structured approach, alternating between low and high carb days on a weekly or biweekly basis, while others may prefer a more intuitive approach based on hunger cues, energy levels, and performance.

Incorporating carb cycling into a low carb diet requires strategic food choices during both low and high carb days. On low carb days, focus on nutrient-dense, low carb foods such as lean proteins, non-starchy vegetables, healthy fats, and small portions of low glycemic index carbohydrates. On high carb days, prioritize complex carbohydrates like whole grains, legumes, fruits, and starchy vegetables to replenish glycogen stores and support energy levels.

While carb cycling can enhance fat loss and metabolic flexibility, it's essential to approach it with caution and awareness of individual tolerance and preferences. Some people may thrive on a structured carb cycling regimen, while others may find it challenging to adhere to or experience adverse effects such as cravings, fatigue, or disruptions in mood and energy levels. Experimentation and self-awareness are key to finding the right approach that balances fat loss goals with overall health and well-being.

Carb cycling can be a potent strategy for enhancing fat loss within the framework of a low carb diet. By strategically alternating between low and high carb days, individuals can optimize fat burning, preserve muscle mass, and improve metabolic flexibility. However, it's essential to approach carb cycling with careful planning, awareness of individual responses, and a focus on nutrient-dense food choices to maximize its effectiveness while supporting overall health and well-being.

CONCLUSION

In conclusion, embarking on a low carb diet journey is not just about restricting carbohydrates; it's about embracing a lifestyle centered around wholesome, nutrient-dense foods that nourish the body and support long-term health and well-being. Throughout this exploration of low carb eating, we've delved into the fundamentals of understanding macronutrients, mastering the art of reading food labels, and even delving into advanced strategies like carb cycling.

Understanding macronutrients—carbohydrates, proteins, and fats—has provided a foundation for making informed food choices that align with low carb principles. By prioritizing high-quality proteins, healthy fats, and fibrous vegetables while minimizing sugars and starches, individuals can optimize their nutritional intake and promote metabolic health.

Reading food labels for carb content has empowered beginners to navigate the complexities of managing carbohydrate intake more effectively. By focusing on net carbs, considering fiber and sugar content, and paying attention to serving sizes, individuals can make choices that support their low carb goals while ensuring overall nutritional balance.

Advanced strategies like carb cycling offer an additional tool for enhancing fat loss and metabolic flexibility within the context of a low carb diet. By strategically alternating between low and high carb days, individuals can optimize fat burning, preserve muscle mass, and prevent metabolic adaptation, all while enjoying a diverse range of foods that nourish the body and support overall health.

Ultimately, the success of a low carb diet hinges on more than just the foods we eat—it's about embracing a mindset of balance, mindfulness, and self-awareness. It's about listening to our bodies, honoring our hunger and satiety cues, and finding joy in the process of nourishing ourselves with foods that support our health and vitality.

As we conclude this journey through the world of low carb eating, let us remember that it's not just about the destination—it's about the journey itself. It's about the small victories, the lessons learned, and the growth experienced along the way. Whether you're just beginning your low carb journey or are well on your way to achieving your goals, may this newfound knowledge empower you to make choices that support your health, happiness, and well-being for years to come.